American
Red Cross

# COMMUNITY
# FIRST AID &
# SAFETY

## Important certification information

American Red Cross certificates may be issued upon successful completion of a training program that uses this textbook as an integral part of the
course. By itself, the text material does not constitute comprehensive
Red Cross training. In order to issue American Red Cross certificates,
your instructor must be authorized by the American Red Cross and must
follow prescribed policies and procedures. Make certain that you have at-
tended a course authorized by the Red Cross. Ask your instructor about
receiving American Red Cross certification, or contact your local chapter
for more information.

**American Red Cross**

# COMMUNITY
# FIRST AID &
# SAFETY

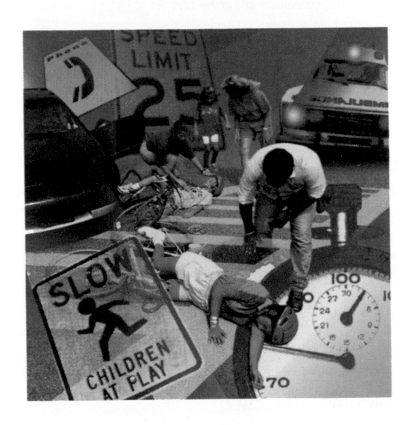

StayWell

# StayWell

This participant's textbook is an integral part of American Red Cross training. By itself, it does not constitute complete and comprehensive training.

The emergency care procedures outlined in this book reflect the standard of knowledge and accepted emergency practices in the United States at the time this book was published. It is the reader's responsibility to stay informed of changes in the emergency care procedures.

The care steps for CPR outlined within this product are consistent with the Guidelines 2000 for Emergency Cardiopulmonary Resuscitation and Emergency Cardiovascular Care.

Printed in the United States of America.

Composition by Graphic World
Printing/Binding by Banta

**StayWell**
**780 Township Line Road**
**Yardley, PA  19067**

**Library of Congress Cataloging in Publication Data**

Community First Aid & Safety / American Red Cross.
     p.  cm.
   ISBN 1-58480-105-0
   1.  First aid in illness and injury.     I.  American Red Cross.
RC86.7.C644   1993                 92-585
616.02′52—dc20
                                                    CIP

       04 05 / 9 8 7 6 5 4 3

# FOOTNOTES

1. McCaig L. National Hospital Ambulatory Medical Care Survey: 1998 Emergency Department Summary. *Adv Data* 10 May 2000; 313.

2. Burt CW and Fingerhut LA. Injury Visits to Hospital Emergency Departments: United States, 1992-95. Vital Health Statistics 13 (131). DHHS publication no. 98-1792. Hyattsville, MD: National Center for Health Statistics, 1998.

3. National Center for Health Statistics, Centers for Disease Control and Prevention. *National Mortality Data,* 1997. Hyattsville, MD: NCHS, 1998.

4. American Heart Association. *2001 Heart and Stroke Statistical Update.* Dallas, TX: American Heart Association, 2000.

5. American Stroke Association. What Is Stroke? Available at **http://www.strokeassociation.org** Accessed on February 8, 2001.

6. Mejicano GC and Maki DG. Infections Acquired During Cardiopulmonary Resuscitation: Estimating the Risk and Defining Strategies for Prevention. *Ann Intern Med* 15 November 1998;129:813-828.

7. American Red Cross Advisory Council on First Aid and Safety, American Red Cross. Advisory Statement on Epinephrine Administration by Lay Rescuers. Available at **http://www.redcross.org** Go to the *Health and Safety Services* section and click on *Resources.* Accessed on February 22, 2001.

8. American Red Cross Advisory Council on First Aid and Safety, American Red Cross. Advisory Statement on Use of the Heimlich Maneuver First Not Recommended in Near-drowning Victims. Available at **http://www.redcross.org** Go to the Health and Safety Services section and click on Resources. Accessed on February 22, 2001.

9. American Heart Association. *2001 Heart and Stroke Statistical Update.* Dallas, TX: American Heart Association, 2000.

10. Centers for Disease Control and Prevention as quoted in Cardiac Arrests on Rise in Young. *Nursing Spectrum;* 11(7DC): April 2, 2001.

11. National Heart, Lung and Blood Institute, National Institutes of Health. 2000. Available at **http://www.nhlbi.nih.gov** Accessed on February 12, 2001.

12. American Heart Association. *2001 Heart and Stroke Statistical Update.* Dallas, TX: American Heart Association, 2000.

13. American Heart Association. 2000 Guidelines for Cardiopulmonary Resuscitation and Emergency Cardiovascular Care. *Circulation;* 102(8): August 22, 2000.

14. American Heart Association. 2000 Guidelines for Cardiopulmonary Resuscitation and Emergency Cardiovascular Care. *Circulation;* 102(8): August 22, 2000.

15. American Heart Association. *2001 Heart and Stroke Statistical Update.* Dallas, TX: American Heart Association, 2000.

16. American Heart Association. *2001 Heart and Stroke Statistical Update.* Dallas, TX: American Heart Association, 2000.

17. American Stroke Association. What Is Stroke? Available at **http://www.strokeassociation.org** Accessed on February 8, 2001.

18. National Stroke Association. All About Stroke. Available at **www.stroke.org** Accessed on February 8, 2001.

19. National Institute of Neurological Disorders and Stroke, National Institutes of Health. NINDS Alzheimer's Disease Information Page. Available at **http://www.ninds.nih.gov/health_and_medical/disorders/alzheimersdisease_doc.html** Accessed on February 6, 2001.

20. American Academy of Family Physicians. Stroke: Warning Signs and Tips on Prevention. Available at **http://familydoctor.org** Accessed on February 8, 2001.

21. American Academy of Family Physicians. Stroke: Warning Signs and Tips on Prevention. Available at **http://familydoctor.org** Accessed on February 8, 2001.

22. American Heart Association. *2001 Heart and Stroke Statistical Update.* Dallas, TX: American Heart Association, 2000.

23. National Safe KIDS Campaign. Available at **http://www.safekids.org** Accessed on March 20, 2001.

24. McCaig L. National Hospital Ambulatory Medical Care Survey: 1998 Emergency Department Summary. *Adv Data* 10 May 2000; 313.

25. National Safety Council. *Injury Facts™,* 2000 Edition. Itasca, IL: 2000.

26. American Red Cross Advisory Council on First Aid and Safety, American Red Cross. Advisory Statement on Epinephrine Administration by Lay Rescuers. Available at **http://www.redcross.org** Go to the *Health and Safety Services* section and click on *Resources.* Accessed on February 22, 2001.

27. Sudden Infant Death Syndrome Alliance. Facts About Sudden Infant Death Syndrome. Available at **http://www.sidsalliance.org** Accessed on February 7, 2001.

28. Sudden Infant Death Syndrome Alliance. Facts About Sudden Infant Death Syndrome. Available at **http://www.sidsalliance.org** Accessed on February 7, 2001.

29. Jeffery HE, Megevand A, Page HD as quoted by Sudden Infant Death Syndrome Network. Available at **http://www.sids-network.org/experts/prone-risk.html** Accessed on February 7, 2001.

30. Sudden Infant Death Syndrome Alliance. Facts About Sudden Infant Death Syndrome. Available at **http://www.sidsalliance.org** Accessed on February 7, 2001.

31. National Safety Council. *Injury Facts™,* 2000 Edition. Itasca, IL: 2000.

32. Burn Foundation. Burn Incidence and Treatment in the United States: 1999 Fact Sheet. Available at **http://www.burnfoundation.org** Accessed on February 20, 2001.

33. National Fire Protection Association. NFPA Fact Sheet on Home Fire Statistics. Available at **http://www.nfpa.org** Accessed on February 20, 2001.

34. Burt CW and Fingerhut LA. Injury Visits to Hospital Emergency Departments: United States, 1992-95. Vital Health Statistics 13 (131). DHHS publication no. 98-1792. Hyattsville, MD: National Center for Health Statistics, 1998.

35. National Criminal Justice Reference Service, US Department of Justice. Available at **http://www.ncjrs.org** Accessed on April 19, 2001.

36. National Center for Injury Prevention and Control, Centers for Disease Control and Prevention. Overall Firearm Deaths and Rates Per 100,000. Available at **http://www.cdc.gov/ncipc/data/us9794/0fam.html** Accessed on February 13, 2001.

37. National Center for Injury Prevention and Control, Centers for Disease Control and Prevention. Overall Firearm Deaths and Rates Per 100,000. Available at **http://www.cdc.gov/ncipc/data/us9794/0fam.html** Accessed on February 13, 2001.

38. The National Clearinghouse for Alcohol and Drug Information. Blood Alcohol Concentration. Available at **http://www.health.org/govpubs/phd627/blood.htm** Accessed on February 12, 2001.

39. National Center for Statistics and Analysis, National Highway Traffic Safety Administration. Available at **http://www.nhtsa.dot.gov/people/ncsa** Accessed on January 29, 2001.

40. Stinson FS and DeBakey SF. 1992. Alcohol-Related Mortality in the United States, 1979-1988. *British Journal of Addiction* 87:777-783.

41. Stinson FS, Dufour MC, Steffens RA and DeBakey SF. 1993. Alcohol-Related Mortality in the United States, 1979-1989. *Alcohol Health and Research* World 17:251-260.

42. American Trauma Society. Available at **http://www.amtrauma.org** Accessed on March 6, 2001.

43. National Safety Council. *Injury Facts™,* 2000 Edition. Itasca, IL: 2000.

44. National Center for Statistics and Analysis, National Highway Traffic Safety Administration. Available at **http://www.nhtsa.dot.gov/people/ncsa** Accessed on January 29, 2001.

45. National Center for Statistics and Analysis, National Highway Traffic Safety Administration. Available at **http://www.nhtsa.dot.gov/people/ncsa** Accessed on January 29, 2001.

46. National Center for Injury Prevention and Control, Centers for Disease Control and Prevention. Overall Firearm Deaths and Rates Per 100,000. Available at **http://www.cdc.gov/ncipc/data/us9794/0fam.html** Accessed on February 13, 2001.

47. National Center for Injury Prevention and Control, Centers for Disease Control and Prevention. Falls and Hip Fractures Among Older Adults. Available at **http://www.cdc.gov/ncipc** Accessed on February 12, 2001.

48. National Safety Council. *Injury Facts™*, 2000 Edition. Itasca, IL: 2000.

49. National Safety Council. *Injury Facts™*, 2000 Edition. Itasca, IL: 2000.

50. National Center for Injury Prevention and Control, Centers for Disease Control and Prevention. Scientific Data, Surveillance, & Injury Statistics. Available at **http://www.cdc.gov/ncipc/ osp.data.htm** Accessed on February 12-14, 2001.

51. National Center for Injury Prevention and Control, Centers for Disease Control and Prevention. Scientific Data, Surveillance, & Injury Statistics. Available at **http://www.cdc.gov/ncipc/ osp.data.htm** Accessed on February 12-14, 2001.

52. Occupational Health and Safety Administration, US Department of Labor. OSHA Directives CPL 2–2.44D—Enforcement Procedures for the Occupational Exposure to Bloodborne Pathogens, Nov. 5, 1999.

53. American Academy of Pediatric Dentistry. Available at **http://www.aapd.org** Accessed on March 8, 2001.

54. Burn Foundation. Burn Incidence and Treatment in the United States: 1999 Fact Sheet. Available at **http://www. burnfoundation.org** Accessed on February 20, 2001.

55. Kessler E. *The Thunderstorm in Human Affairs*. Norman, OK: University of Oklahoma, 1983.

56. National Center for Injury Prevention and Control, Centers for Disease Control and Prevention. Scientific Data, Surveillance, & Injury Statistics. Available at **http://www.cdc.gov/ncipc/ osp.data.htm** Accessed on February 12-14, 2001.

57. National Athletic Trainers Association. NATA Recommendations for Lightning Safety. NATA News November 2000; Insert.

58. Burn Foundation. Burn Incidence and Treatment in the United States: 1999 Fact Sheet. Available at **http://www. burnfoundation.org** Accessed on February 20, 2001.

59. American Academy of Dermatology. Going to Summer Camp This Year? Then Read On...Fry Now, Pay Later. Available at **http://www.aad.org/SkinCancerNews/SafeSunTips/ SummerCamp.html** Accessed on February 12, 2001.

60. American Academy of Ophthalmology as quoted in Healthy Tips for Summer. *The Saturday Evening Post:* July, 2000.

61. National Osteoporosis Foundation. Fast Facts on Osteoporosis. Available at **http://www.nof.org** Accessed on February 15, 2001.

62. National Center for Injury Prevention and Control, Centers for Disease Control and Prevention. Falls and Hip Fractures Among Older Adults. Available at **http://www.cdc.gov/ncipc** Accessed on February 12, 2001.

63. National Spinal Cord Injury Association. Spinal Cord Injury Statistics. Available at **http://www.spinalcord.org/ resource/Factsheets/factsheet2.html** Accessed on February 20, 2001.

64. National Center for Injury Prevention and Control, Centers for Disease Control and Prevention. Scientific Data, Surveillance, & Injury Statistics. Available at **http://www.cdc.gov/ncipc/ osp.data.htm** Accessed on February 12-14, 2001.

65. Epilepsy Foundation of America. Epilepsy: A Report to the Nation. Available at **http://www.efa.org/epusa/nation/nation.html** Accessed on February 26, 2001.

66. American Diabetes Association. Available at **http://www. diabetes.org/ada/facts.asp** Accessed on February 2, 2001.

67. American Diabetes Association. Available at **http://www. diabetes.org/ada/facts.asp** Accessed on February 2, 2001.

68. Juvenile Diabetes Foundation. Get the Facts: Type 1 Diabetes Fact Sheet. Available at **http://www.jdf.org** Accessed on February 8, 2001.

69. American Diabetes Association. Available at **http://www. diabetes.org/ada/facts.asp** Accessed on February 2, 2001.

70. American Diabetes Association. Available at **http://www. diabetes.org/ada/facts.asp** Accessed on February 2, 2001.

71. American Red Cross Advisory Council on First Aid and Safety, American Red Cross. Advisory Statement on Oral Glucose (Sugar) Administration by Lay Rescuers. Available at **http://www. redcross.org** Go to the *Health and Safety Services* section and click on *Resources.* Accessed on February 22, 2001.

72. Epilepsy Foundation of America. Seizure Recognition and First Aid Brochure, 2000.

73. Litovitz TL, Klein-Schwartz W, Caravati EM, Youniss J, Crouch B, Lee S. 1998 Annual Report of the American Association of Poison Control Centers Toxic Exposure Surveillance System. *Amer J Emer Med* 1999;17(5):435-87.

74. National Center for Injury Prevention and Control, Centers for Disease Control and Prevention. Facts About Poisoning. Available at **http://www.cdc.gov/ncipc** Accessed on February 13, 2001.

75. National Capital Poison Center. 1999. Available at **http://www.poison.org** Accessed on March 19, 2001.

76. Centers for Disease Control and Prevention. Facts About Lyme Disease. Available at **http://www.cdc.gov/od/oc/media/ fact/lyme.htm** Accessed on February 7, 2001.

77. National Institute of Allergy and Infectious Diseases, National Institute of Health. Lyme Disease-The Facts, The Challenge. Available at **http://www.niaid.nih.gov/publications/ lyme/textonly.htm** Accessed on February 13, 2001.

78. Palm Beach Herpetological Society in Cooperation with the Florida Cooperative Extension Service, Institute of Food and Agricultural Sciences, University of Florida. Venomous Snake Bite. Available at **http://www.cdc.gov.niosh/nasd/docs/ as31600.html** Accessed on February 20, 2001.

79. National Center for Health Statistics, Centers for Disease Control and Prevention. *Health, United States, 1999: With Health and Aging Chartbook.* Hyattsville, MD: 1999.

80. National Institute of Neurological Disorders and Stroke, National Institutes of Health. Brain Attack. Available at **http://www.ninds.nih.gov** Accessed on February 8, 2001.

81. Alzheimer's Association. General Statistics/Demographics. September 12, 2000. Available at **http://www.alz.org** Accessed on February 6, 2001.

# REFERENCES

American Academy of Dermatology. Facts About Sunscreens. 1991. Available at **http://www.aad.org** Accessed on February 12, 2001.

Mothers Against Drunk Driving. Available at **http://www.madd.org/**Accessed on March 30, 2001.

National Center for HIV, STD and TB Prevention, Centers for Disease Control and Prevention. Available at **http://www.cdc.gov/hiv/ hivinfo/nah.htm** Accessed on April 19, 2001.

National Maternal Child Health Clearinghouse. Available at **http://www.nmchc.org** Accessed on January 30, 2001.

National Pesticide Telecommunications Network. Available at **http://nptn.orsted.edu** Accessed on February 28, 2001.

Students Against Destructive Decisions. Available at **www.saddonline.com** Accessed on March 30, 2001.

US Consumer Product Safety Commission. Available at **http://www.uscpsc.gov** Accessed on January 30, 2001.

# ABOUT THIS COURSE

People need to know what to do in an emergency before medical help arrives. Since you may be faced with an emergency in your lifetime, it is important that you know how to recognize an emergency and how to respond. The intent of this course is to help lay responders feel more confident in their ability to act appropriately in the event of an emergency.

After you complete this course, you will be able to—
* Identify ways to prevent injury or illness.
* Recognize when an emergency has occurred.
* Follow three emergency action steps in any emergency.
* Provide basic care for injury or sudden illness until the victim can receive emergency medical help.

To help you achieve this goal, you will read information in this manual, view a series of video segments and participate in a number of learning activities designed to increase your knowledge and skills.

In addition, this course emphasizes the value of a safe and healthy lifestyle. It attempts to alert you to behavior and situations that contribute to your risk of injury or illness and to motivate you to take precautions and make any necessary lifestyle changes.

This manual contains material you learn in class in a form you can keep and refer to whenever you wish. Information is highlighted and condensed in lists to make it easy for you to identify the critical points and to refresh your memory quickly. Photos, drawings, graphs and tables also present information in an easy-to-find form. Skill sheets give step-by-step directions for performing the skills taught in the course. Questionnaires provide a way for you to evaluate certain risks in your lifestyle. Informational sidebars enhance the material you have learned.

You may be taking this course because you feel a need to learn what to do if faced with an emergency. You also may be taking this course because of a job (whether as an employee or volunteer) requirement specifying that you complete training and achieve a specific level of competency on both skill and written evaluations. In either case, the American Red Cross provides a course completion certificate. You will be eligible to receive a certificate if you—
* Perform required skills competently and demonstrate the ability to make appropriate decisions for care.
* Pass a final written exam(s) with a score of 80 percent or higher for each section.

If you do not have a requirement to achieve a specific level of competency on both skill and written evaluations, you will not need a course completion certificate.

# HEALTH PRECAUTIONS AND GUIDELINES DURING TRAINING

The American Red Cross has trained millions of people in first aid and cardiopulmonary resuscitation (CPR), using manikins as training aids. According to the Centers for Disease Control and Prevention (CDC), there has never been a documented case of any disease caused by bacteria, fungi or viruses transmitted through the use of training aids, such as manikins used for CPR.

The American Red Cross follows widely accepted guidelines for cleaning and decontaminating training manikins. **If these guidelines are adhered to, the risk of any kind of disease transmission during training is extremely low.**

To help minimize the risk of disease transmission, you should follow some basic health precautions and guidelines while participating in training. You should take precautions if you have a condition that would increase your risk or other participants' risk of exposure to infections. Request a separate training manikin if you—

- Have an acute condition, such as a cold, a sore throat, or cuts or sores on your hands or around your mouth.
- Have had a positive blood test for hepatitis B surface antigen (HBsAG), indicating that you are currently infected with the hepatitis B virus.*
- Know you have a chronic infection indicated by long-term seropositivity (long-term positive blood tests) for hepatitis B surface antigen (HBsAG)* or a positive blood test to anti-HIV (that is, a positive test for antibodies to HIV, the virus that causes AIDS).
- Have had a positive blood test for hepatitis C.
- Have a condition that makes you unusually likely to get an infection.

To obtain information about testing for individual health status, go to: www.cdc.gov/ncidod/diseases/hepatitis/c/faq.htm

*A person with hepatitis B infection will test positive for the hepatitis B surface antigen (HBsAG). Most persons infected with hepatitis B will get better within a period of time. However, some hepatitis B infections will become chronic and linger for much longer. These persons will continue to test positive for HBsAG. Their decision to participate in CPR training should be guided by their health-care provider.

After a person has an acute hepatitis B infection, he or she will no longer test positive for the surface antigen but will test positive for the hepatitis B antibody. A positive test for the hepatitis B antibody (anti-HBs) should not be confused with a positive test for the hepatitis B surface antigen (HBsAG).

**If you decide you should have your own manikin, ask your instructor if he or she can provide one for you to use.** You will not be asked to explain why in your request. The manikin will not be used by anyone else until it has been cleaned according to the recommended end-of-class decontamination procedures. The number of manikins available for class use is limited. Therefore, the more advance notice you give, the more likely it is that you will be provided a separate manikin.

In addition to taking precautions regarding manikins, you can further protect yourself and other participants from infection by following these guidelines:

- Wash your hands thoroughly before participating in class activities.
- Do not eat, drink, use tobacco products or chew gum during classes when manikins are used.
- Clean the manikin properly after use. For some manikins, this means vigorously wiping the manikin's face and the inside of its mouth with a clean gauze pad soaked with either a solution of $\frac{1}{2}$ cup liquid chlorine bleach per gallon of tap water (sodium hypochlorite and tap water) or rubbing alcohol. The surfaces should remain wet for at least 30 seconds before they are wiped dry with a second piece of clean, absorbent material. For other manikins, it means changing the rubber face. Your instructor will provide you with instructions for cleaning the type of manikin used in your class. Follow the guidelines provided by your instructor when practicing skills such as clearing a blocked airway with your finger.

Training in first aid and CPR requires physical activity. If you have a medical condition or disability that will prevent you from taking part in the practice sessions, please let your instructor know so that accommodations can be made.

# CONTENTS

**6** First Aid and Disease Transmission

**21** What Happens When You Call EMS

Why did you say you'd get to the party by seven o'clock? It's a good thing you stopped at the convenience store now and not later. Only a couple of things to buy. Why are all those people standing around over there? Oh no! It's the person who works here... You leave the car and see the young man lying on his back, looking dazed and holding his head. Even though a crowd has gathered, no one is helping him. They are just looking at each other. He needs help from some-one. That someone could be you.

**If not YOU...**
**Who?**

GET INVOLVED

I f placed in the above situation, would you step forward to help? "I hope I never have to," is what you are probably saying to yourself. However, given the number of injuries and sudden illnesses that occur in the United States each year, you might well have to deal with an emergency situation someday.

Consider the following:
- Over 37 million injury-related visits[1] were made to U.S. hospital emergency departments in 1998; injuries resulted in almost 90,000 deaths.[2]

- Previously, infectious diseases caused the greatest risk to the health and well-being of children, but now, unintentional injuries cause most childhood deaths.
- Injuries also cause millions of heart-stopping moments each year. In fact, injuries are the leading cause of death and disability in children and young adults.[3]
- More than 60 million people in the United States have cardiovascular disease. Cardiovascular disease causes about 1 million deaths in the United States each year.[4] That accounts for over 40 percent of all U.S. deaths that occur annually!
- Over 600,000 Americans have strokes each year and more than 160,000 Americans die annually from stroke.[5]

Each time a person is injured or experiences a sudden illness, such as a heart attack or a stroke, someone has to do something to help. You may find yourself in the position of having to provide help someday.

Everyone should know what to do in an emergency. You should know who to call and what care to provide. Providing care involves giving first aid until emergency medical help arrives. Everyone should know first aid, but even if you have not had any first aid training you can still help in an emergency.

▼

# Everyone Should Know What to Do in an Emergency...

# Everyone Should Know First Aid.

Calling 9-1-1 or the local emergency number is the most important step you can take in an emergency. The sooner emergency medical help arrives, the better a person's chance of surviving a life-threatening emergency. You play a major role in making the emergency medical services (EMS) system work effectively. The EMS system is a network of police, fire and medical personnel, as well as other community resources.

Your role in the EMS system includes four basic steps:
1. *Recognize* that an emergency exists.

Accidents 46,464

Cancer 24,562

Heart Disease 19,006

Suicide 16,661

Homicide 14,819

**Leading Causes of Death**
**ages 0 to 44**

National Safety Council Tabulations of 1998 National Center for Health Statistics Mortality Data.

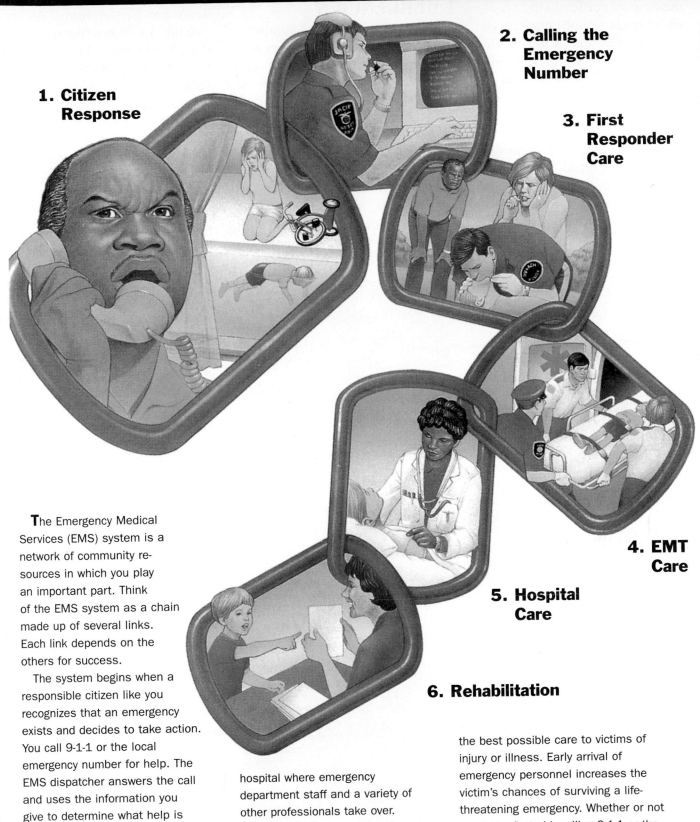

**1. Citizen Response**

**2. Calling the Emergency Number**

**3. First Responder Care**

**4. EMT Care**

**5. Hospital Care**

**6. Rehabilitation**

The Emergency Medical Services (EMS) system is a network of community resources in which you play an important part. Think of the EMS system as a chain made up of several links. Each link depends on the others for success.

The system begins when a responsible citizen like you recognizes that an emergency exists and decides to take action. You call 9-1-1 or the local emergency number for help. The EMS dispatcher answers the call and uses the information you give to determine what help is needed. A team of emergency personnel gives care at the scene and transports the victim to the hospital where emergency department staff and a variety of other professionals take over.

Ideally, a victim will move through each link in the EMS system. All the links should work together to provide the best possible care to victims of injury or illness. Early arrival of emergency personnel increases the victim's chances of surviving a life-threatening emergency. Whether or not you know first aid, calling 9-1-1 or the local emergency number is the most important action you can take.

2. *Decide* to act.
3. *Call* 9-1-1 or the local emergency number for help.
4. *Provide* care until help arrives.

Of course, steps 3 and 4 will not happen if you do not take steps 1 and 2. By recognizing an emergency and taking action to help, you give injured or ill persons the best chance for survival. Know your local emergency number. The rapid arrival of emergency medical help increases the victim's chances of surviving a life-threatening emergency.

# RECOGNIZING EMERGENCIES

Emergencies can happen to anyone and they can happen anywhere. But before you can give help, you must be able to recognize an emergency. You may realize that an emergency has occurred only if something unusual attracts your attention. For example, you may become aware of unusual noises, sights, odors and appearances or behaviors.

Noises that may signal an emergency include screaming or calls for help; breaking glass, crashing metal or screeching tires; a change in the sound made by machinery or equipment; or sudden, loud noises, like those made by collapsing buildings or falling ladders or when a person falls.

Signals of an emergency that you may see include a person lying motionless, spilled chemicals, fallen boxes, a power failure or downed electrical wires, smoke or fire.

Many odors are part of our everyday lives; for example, gasoline fumes at the gas station, the smell of chlorine at a swimming pool and the smell of chemicals at a refinery. However, when these are stronger than usual, there may be an emergency. Also, an unusual odor may mean something is wrong. Put your own safety first. Leave the area if there is an unusual or very strong odor, since some fumes are poisonous.

It may be difficult to tell if someone is behaving strangely or if something is wrong, especially if you do not know the person. Some actions leave little doubt that something might be wrong. For example, if you see someone suddenly collapse or slip and fall, you have a fairly good idea that the person might need some help.

Other signals of a possible emergency might not be as easy to recognize. They include signals of trouble breathing, confused behavior, unusual skin color, signs of pain and discomfort such as clutching the chest or throat, being doubled over or facial expressions indicating something is wrong.

Sometimes it is obvious that something is wrong; at other times it is more difficult to be sure. For example, a person having a heart attack may clutch his

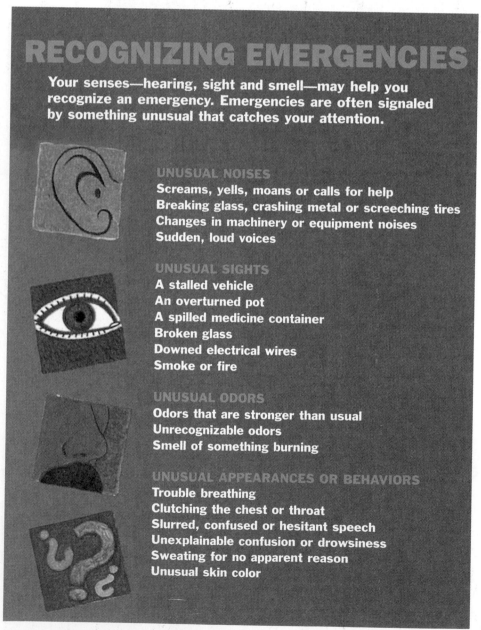

## RECOGNIZING EMERGENCIES

**Your senses—hearing, sight and smell—may help you recognize an emergency. Emergencies are often signaled by something unusual that catches your attention.**

### UNUSUAL NOISES
Screams, yells, moans or calls for help
Breaking glass, crashing metal or screeching tires
Changes in machinery or equipment noises
Sudden, loud voices

### UNUSUAL SIGHTS
A stalled vehicle
An overturned pot
A spilled medicine container
Broken glass
Downed electrical wires
Smoke or fire

### UNUSUAL ODORS
Odors that are stronger than usual
Unrecognizable odors
Smell of something burning

### UNUSUAL APPEARANCES OR BEHAVIORS
Trouble breathing
Clutching the chest or throat
Slurred, confused or hesitant speech
Unexplainable confusion or drowsiness
Sweating for no apparent reason
Unusual skin color

or her chest, begin to perspire and have trouble breathing. Another heart attack victim may only feel mild chest discomfort and not give any obvious signals of distress. The important thing is to recognize that an emergency might have occurred.

## DECIDING TO ACT

Once you recognize an emergency has occurred, you must decide whether to help or how you can help. There are many ways you can help in an emergency. *In order to help, you must act.*

▼

# There are Many Ways to Help in an Emergency. In Order to Help, You Must Act.

Whether or not you have had first aid training, being faced with an emergency will probably cause you to have mixed feelings. Besides wanting to help, you may have other feelings that make you hesitate or back away from the situation. These feelings are personal and very real. The decision to act is yours and yours alone.

Sometimes, even though people recognize that what has happened is an emergency, they fail to act. There are many reasons

# What Everyone Should Know About Good Samaritan Laws

Are there laws to protect you when you help in an emergency situation?

Yes, most states have enacted Good Samaritan laws. These laws give legal protection to people who gratuitously provide emergency care to ill or injured persons.

When a citizen responds to an emergency and acts as a *reasonable* and *prudent* person would under the same conditions, Good Samaritan immunity generally prevails. For example, a reasonable and prudent person would—

- Move a victim only if the victim's life was endangered.
- Ask a conscious victim for permission before giving care.
- Check the victim for life-threatening conditions before providing further care.
- Summon emergency medical personnel to the scene by calling 9-1-1 or the local emergency number.
- Continue to provide care until more highly trained personnel arrive.

Good Samaritan laws were developed to encourage people to help others in emergency situations. They require that the "Good Samaritan" use common sense and a reasonable level of skill, not to exceed the scope of the individual's training in emergency situations. They assume each person would do his or her best to save a life or prevent further injury.

Lay responders are rarely sued for helping in an emergency. However, Good Samaritan laws protect the responder from financial responsibility. In cases where an individual lay responder's response was deliberately negligent or reckless or when the responder abandoned the victim after initiating care, the courts have ruled Good Samaritan immunity did not apply.

If you are interested in finding out about your state's Good Samaritan laws, contact a legal professional or check with your local library.

why people do not act in an emergency. The most common factors that influence a person's response include—

- The presence of other people.
- Uncertainty that an emergency really exists.
- Uncertainty about the victim.
- The type of injury or illness.
- Fear of catching a disease.
- Fear of doing something wrong.
- Fear of being sued.

If there are several people standing around, it might not be easy to tell if anyone is providing first aid. Always ask if you can help. Just because there is a crowd does not mean someone is caring for the victim. In fact, you may be the only one there who knows first aid.

Although you may feel embarrassed about coming forward in front of other people, this should not stop you from offering help. Someone has to take action in an emergency and it may have to be you, even though you do not want to become the center of attention. If others are already giving care, ask if you can help.

If there are people around who do not appear to be helping, tell them how to help. You can ask them to call 9-1-1 or the local emergency number, meet the ambulance and direct it to your location, keep the area free of onlookers and traffic or help give care. You might send them for blankets or other supplies.

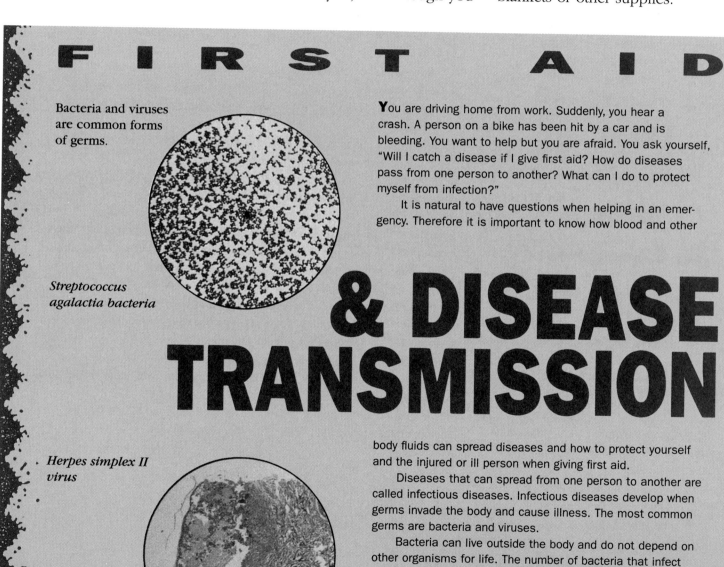

# FIRST AID & DISEASE TRANSMISSION

Bacteria and viruses are common forms of germs.

*Streptococcus agalactia bacteria*

*Herpes simplex II virus*

You are driving home from work. Suddenly, you hear a crash. A person on a bike has been hit by a car and is bleeding. You want to help but you are afraid. You ask yourself, "Will I catch a disease if I give first aid? How do diseases pass from one person to another? What can I do to protect myself from infection?"

It is natural to have questions when helping in an emergency. Therefore it is important to know how blood and other body fluids can spread diseases and how to protect yourself and the injured or ill person when giving first aid.

Diseases that can spread from one person to another are called infectious diseases. Infectious diseases develop when germs invade the body and cause illness. The most common germs are bacteria and viruses.

Bacteria can live outside the body and do not depend on other organisms for life. The number of bacteria that infect humans is really very small, but some can cause serious infections. These can be treated with special medications called antibiotics.

Viruses depend on other organisms to live. Once in the body, they are hard to remove. Few medications can fight viruses. The body's immune system is the number one protection against infection.

# There are Some Simple Things You Can Do to Prevent Disease Transmission.

TAKE PRECAUTIONS

You may wonder how bacteria and viruses spread from one person to another. Well, in situations that require first aid care, some diseases can be transmitted by touching, breathing and biting.

You can become infected if you touch an infected person. This can happen when germs from the person's blood or other body fluids pass into your body through breaks or cuts in your skin or through the lining of your eyes, nose or mouth. Your skin and the lining of your eyes, nose or mouth are protective barriers; when those barriers are broken by even a very small cut or break, germs can pass through. Therefore a greater risk of infection occurs when you touch blood or other body fluids directly. This is the same for a victim, who can be infected by a responder. Using breathing barriers and disposable gloves can reduce the likelihood of infection.

You can also be infected when you touch an object that has been soiled by a person's blood or body fluids. Be careful when handling soiled objects. Sharp objects can cut your skin and spread germs. Avoid touching blood and soiled objects with your bare hands.

Some diseases, such as the common cold, are transmitted by droplets in the air we breathe and through contact with shared objects like spoons, doorknobs and pencils that have been exposed to the droplets. It is possible to become infected by some diseases if you breathe air exhaled by an infected person. Airborne infection can occur during sneezing, coughing, speaking, etc. All of us are exposed to germs every day in our jobs, on the bus or in a crowded restaurant. Fortunately, simply being exposed to these germs is usually not adequate for diseases to be transmitted. Your immune system will help your body fight off these germs and help to protect you from infections.

Animals can spread some diseases through bites. For example, infected dogs, cats, cattle and some wild animals can transmit rabies. A human bite also can cause disease. Contracting a disease from a bite is rare in any situation and

very uncommon when giving first aid. In an emergency situation, it is unlikely that you will be bitten.

Some diseases are spread more easily than others. We all know how quickly the flu can spread from person to person at home or at work. Although these diseases can create discomfort, they are often temporary and are not serious to healthy adults.

Other germs can be more serious, such as hepatitis B virus (HBV), hepatitis C (HCV) virus and the human immunodeficiency virus (HIV), which causes acquired immune deficiency syndrome (AIDS). Although very serious, they are not easily transmitted and are not spread by casual contact, such as shaking hands. The primary way to transmit HBV, HCV or HIV during first aid care is through blood-to-blood contact.

By following some basic guidelines, you can help reduce disease transmission when providing first aid:

- Avoid contact with body fluids when possible.
- Use protective breathing barriers for any emergency situation requiring you to give rescue breaths.
- Place barriers, such as disposable gloves or a clean dry cloth, between the victim's body fluids and yourself.
- Use disposable gloves.
- Cover any cuts, sores, scrapes and skin conditions you may have.
- Do not eat, drink or touch your mouth, nose or eyes when giving first aid.
- Do not touch objects that may be soiled with blood.
- Be prepared by having a first aid kit handy and stocked with protective equipment and supplies.
- Wash your hands with soap and water immediately after providing care to a victim.

Following these guidelines greatly decreases your risk of getting or transmitting an infectious disease. Remember always to give first aid in ways that protect you and the victim from disease transmission.

# You are More Likely to Give Care to a Family Member or a Friend Than to Someone You Don't Know.

Most emergencies happen in or near the home, so you are more likely to give care to a family member or a friend than to someone you do not know. However, this is not always the case. There may be a time when you do not know the victim and feel uneasy about helping a stranger. Sometimes you might not be sure about taking action because of who the victim is. For example, the victim may be much older or much younger than you, be a different gender or race, have a disabling condition, be of a different status at work or be a victim of a crime.

Sometimes people who have been injured or become suddenly ill act strangely or may be hard to deal with. The injury or illness, stress or other factors such as the effects of drugs, alcohol or medications may make people unpleasant or angry. Do not take this behavior personally. If you feel at all threatened by the victim's behavior, leave the immediate area and call 9-1-1 or the local emergency number for help.

Another factor that affects a person's decision to do something in an emergency is the type of injury or illness. An injury or illness may sometimes be very unpleasant. Blood, vomit, unpleasant odors, deformed body parts or torn or burned skin upset almost everyone. You may have to turn away for a moment and take a few deep breaths to get control of your feelings. Then try to provide care. If you still cannot give first aid because of the way the injury looks, you can ensure your safety and the safety of victims and bystanders by making sure you or someone else has called 9-1-1 or the local emergency number.

Disease transmission in a first aid situation is another issue that concerns many people. Today, people worry about the possibility of being infected with a disease while giving first aid. This is especially true as an uninformed response to the AIDS epidemic. However, the actual risk of catching a disease like AIDS when giving first aid is far less than you may think.[6]

Giving first aid does not mean that you will automatically catch a disease. In fact, it is extremely unlikely that you will catch a disease by giving first aid. If you do not have any cuts or sores, your skin protects you as you give first aid. Remember that disease transmission works both ways. You can also pass diseases to the victim if you have any cuts or sores on your own skin.

Emergency situations that involve contact with body fluids, such as blood, have the possibility of transmitting disease. There are simple things you can do to minimize the chance of infection. Always take precautions to prevent direct contact with a victim's body fluids while you are giving first aid. When they are available, use protective barriers, such as disposable gloves, when giving care for a bleeding wound. The victim may even be able to use his or her own hand to help. Afterward, wash your hands thoroughly with soap and warm running water as soon as possible, even if you wore gloves. Tell EMS personnel at the scene and your doctor if you come in direct contact with a victim's body fluids while giving first aid.

People react differently in emergencies. Whether trained in first aid or not, some people are afraid of doing the wrong thing and making matters worse. If you are not sure what to do, call 9-1-1 or the local emergency number. *The worst thing to do is nothing.*

Sometimes people worry that they might be sued for giving first aid. In fact, lawsuits against people who give emergency care at a scene of an accident are highly unusual and rarely successful. Most states have enacted "Good Samaritan" laws. These laws protect people who willingly give first aid without ac-

# FACTS

**ABOUT**

# AIDS

*David A. Wagner/Phototake NYC*

*Human Immunodeficiency Virus*

**The Disease:** AIDS stands for acquired immune deficiency syndrome. It is caused by the human immunodeficiency virus (HIV). When the virus gets into the body, it damages the immune system, the body system that fights infection. Once the virus enters the body, it can grow quietly in the body for months or even years. People infected with HIV might not feel or appear sick. Eventually, the weakened immune system gives way to certain types of infections.

**How the Disease is Transmitted:** The virus enters the body in three basic ways:

- Through direct contact with the bloodstream. Examples of this include contact with blood, semen, vaginal fluids or breast milk of an infected mother.
- Through the mucous membrane linings in the eyes, mouth, throat, rectum and vagina. *Example:* having sex without a latex condom with an HIV-positive person—male or female.
- Through being infected as an unborn child or shortly after birth by an infected mother.

The virus cannot enter through the skin unless there is a cut or break in the skin. Even then, the possibility of infection is very low unless there is direct contact for a lengthy period of time. Saliva is not known to transmit HIV.

**Prevention:** Your behavior can put you at risk for being infected with HIV, HBV and HCV. Sharing needles or having sex without protection (such as condoms) puts you at risk.

**First Aid Precautions:** The likelihood of HIV transmission during a first aid situation is very low. Always give care in ways that protect you and the victim from disease transmission. If possible, wash your hands before and after giving care, even if you wear disposable gloves. Avoid touching or being splashed by another person's body fluids, especially blood. Clean any area of your skin that comes in contact with blood or body fluids. Be prepared with a first aid kit that includes waterless antiseptic hand cleaners and disposable gloves. Always wash your hands with soap and warm running water after giving care.

**Testing:** If you think you have put yourself at risk, get tested. A test that is commonly available will tell whether your body is producing antibodies in response to the virus. If you are not sure whether you should be tested, call your doctor, the public health department, an AIDS service organization or the AIDS hotline listed below and talk to them. In the meantime, don't participate in activities that put you or anyone else at risk.

**Blood Supply:** Since 1985, all donated blood in the United States has been tested for HIV. The risk of becoming infected through a blood transfusion is extremely low.

**Hot Line:** If you have any questions, call the Centers for Disease Control and Prevention (CDC) national AIDS hotline at 1-800-342-2437, 24 hours a day, 7 days a week or the SIDA hotline (Spanish) at 1-800-344-7432, 24 hours a day, 7 days a week. TTY/TDD service is available at 1-800-243-7889, Monday-Friday, 10 a.m.-10 p.m., EST. Or call your local or state health department.

# BE PREPARED

Keep medical information about you and your family in a handy place, such as on the refrigerator door or in your automobile glove compartment.

▼

Keep medical and insurance records up to date.

▼

Find out if your community is served by an emergency 9-1-1 telephone number. If it is not, look up the numbers for the police, fire department and EMS. Find out the number for the poison control center. Emergency numbers are usually listed in the front of the telephone book. Teach everyone in your home how and when to use these numbers.

▼

Keep emergency telephone numbers in a handy place, such as by the telephone or in the first aid kit. Include home and work numbers of family members and friends who can help. Be sure to keep both lists current.

▼

Keep a first aid kit handy in your home, automobile, workplace and recreation area.

▼

Learn and practice first aid skills.

▼

Learn how to use an automated external defibrillator (AED) for victims of sudden cardiac arrest.

▼

Make sure your house or apartment number is easy to read. Numerals are easier to read than spelled-out numbers.

▼

Wear a medical alert tag if you have a potentially serious medical condition, such as epilepsy, diabetes, heart disease or allergies.

cepting anything in return. So you can help without worrying about lawsuits.

Your decision to act in an emergency should be guided by your own values and by your knowledge of the risks that may be present. Your decision to act might not involve giving first aid. However, it should at least involve calling 9-1-1 or the local emergency number to get emergency medical help.

## PREPARING FOR EMERGENCIES

If you are prepared for unforeseen emergencies, you can help ensure that care begins as soon as possible for yourself, your family and your fellow citizens. If you are trained in first aid, you can give help that can save a life in the first few minutes of an emergency. First aid can be the difference between

life and death. Often it does make the difference between complete recovery and permanent disability.

By knowing what to do, you will be better able to manage your fears and overcome barriers to action. The most important things are to recognize that an emergency has occurred and to call 9-1-1 or the local emergency number. Then give first aid until emergency medical help arrives.

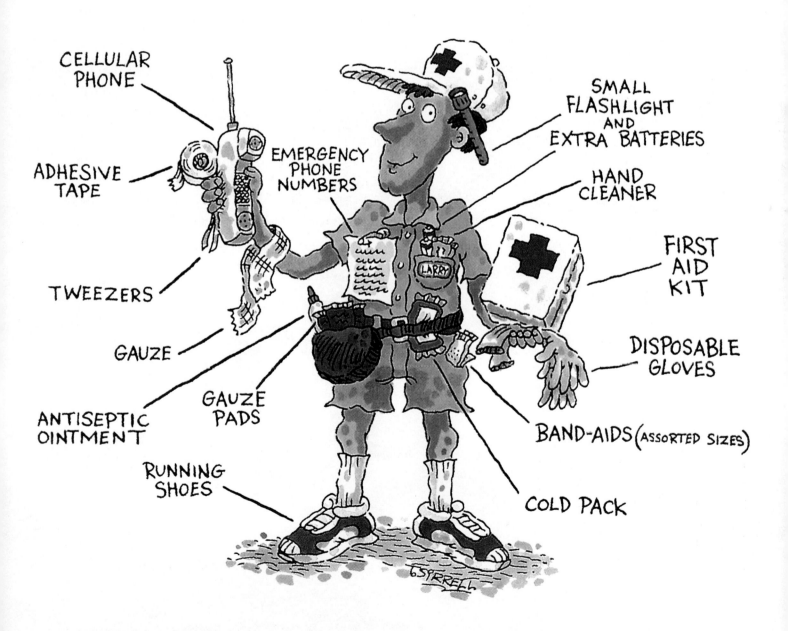

CELLULAR PHONE

ADHESIVE TAPE

TWEEZERS

GAUZE

ANTISEPTIC OINTMENT

GAUZE PADS

RUNNING SHOES

EMERGENCY PHONE NUMBERS

SMALL FLASHLIGHT AND EXTRA BATTERIES

HAND CLEANER

FIRST AID KIT

DISPOSABLE GLOVES

BAND-AIDS (ASSORTED SIZES)

COLD PACK

# TAKING ACTION

## Emergency Action Steps

It's 9:30 on a Saturday morning. The sudden sounds outside are close together but very clear—a screech of brakes, a thud and a shrill scream. You are out the door and onto the sidewalk before you have time to think about it. Maria and Rose had been playing out there!

People are running from all over. Your eyes take it in—the twisted bike, the van in the middle of the street and the child lying on the pavement. At least he's alive; he's moaning and crying. His left leg looks funny and there's blood on the pavement. A man is staring at the boy. "He just came out of nowhere," he stammers. "All of the sudden, there he was, right in front of the van." The boy is obviously hurt. What should you do?

So far, you have learned that you can make a difference in an emergency. You may even save a life. You now know how to recognize an emergency. You have learned that the worst thing you can do is nothing and deciding to get involved can be hard for anyone—not just you. You also know some things you can do to help.

Even so, when an emergency happens, you may feel confused. However, you can train yourself to stay calm and think before you act. Ask yourself, "What do I need to do? What is the best help I can give?" To answer these questions, you should know three basic steps you can take in any emergency:

- *Check* the scene and the victim.
- *Call* 9-1-1 or the local emergency number.
- *Care* for the victim.

## CHECK

Before you can help the victim, you must make sure the scene is safe for you and any bystanders. You also need some information. Look the scene over and try to answer these questions:
1. Is the scene safe?

Don't put yourself in danger ... dead or injured heroes are no help to anyone!

2. What happened?
3. How many victims are there?
4. Can bystanders help?

Check for anything that might make the scene unsafe. Examples include spilled chemicals, traffic, fire, escaping steam, downed electrical lines, smoke, extreme weather and poisonous gas. If these or other dangers threaten, do not go near the victim. Stay at a safe distance and call 9-1-1 or the local emergency number immediately.

If the scene is still unsafe after you call, stay away from the victim. Do not put yourself in danger. Dead or injured heroes are no

help to anyone! Leave dangerous situations to professionals like fire fighters and police who have the training and equipment to deal with them. Once they make the scene safe, you can offer to help.

Try to find out what happened. Look for clues to what caused the emergency and how the victim might be injured. Nearby objects, such as a fallen ladder, broken glass or a spilled bottle of medicine, may give you information. Your check of the scene may be the only way to tell what happened.

Look carefully for more than one victim. You might not spot

CHECK

CHECK THE SCENE
AND THE VICTIM

everyone at first. If one victim is bleeding or screaming, you might not notice an unconscious victim. It is also easy to overlook an infant or a small child. Once you reach the victim, check the scene again. You may see danger, clues or victims you missed before.

Do not move a seriously injured victim unless there is an immediate danger, such as fire, flood or poisonous gas; you have to reach another victim who may have a more serious injury or illness; or you need to move a victim to provide proper care. If you must move the victim, do it as quickly and carefully as possible. If there is no danger, tell the victim not to move. Tell any bystanders not to move the victim.

You have already learned that the presence of bystanders does not mean that a victim is receiving help. Besides doing what you can for the victim, you can ask bystanders to help. They may be able to tell you what happened or direct you to the nearest telephone. A family member, friend or co-worker who is present may know if the victim has an illness or a medical condition. The victim may be too upset to answer your questions. A child may be especially frightened. Anyone who awakens after having been unconscious for a few minutes may also be frightened. Bystanders can also help comfort the victim and others at the scene. Parents or guardians who are present may be able to calm a frightened child. They can also tell you if a child has a medical condition.

When you reach the victim, you must try to find out what is wrong. Look for signals that may indicate a life-threatening emergency. The first thing you check is whether the victim is conscious.

Sometimes this is obvious. The victim may be able to speak to you and tell you what happened. The victim may be moaning, crying or making some other noise. The victim may be moving around. Talk to the victim to reassure him or her and to learn what you can about what happened.

What if the victim is lying on the ground, silent and not moving? You must find out if the victim is conscious or unconscious. Unconsciousness is a life-threatening emergency. If the victim does not respond to you in any way, assume he or she is unconscious. You must make sure that someone calls 9-1-1 or the local emergency number.

Look for other signals of injuries that are life threatening or may become life threatening: no breathing or trouble breathing, no signs of circulation or severe bleeding.

While you are checking the victim, use your senses of sight, smell and hearing. They will help you notice anything abnormal.

For example, an unusual smell may be caused by a poison. You may see a bruise or a twisted arm or leg. Listen carefully to what the victim says.

## CALL

It is very important that you know your local emergency number. It may be 9-1-1, 0 for an operator, a local number or a special response number where you work. Post your emergency number by the phone at home and at work. If you are using a cellular phone, you must know your location or nearby landmarks. Calling 9-1-1 from a cellular phone is a free call.

Calling for help is often the most important action you can take to help the victim. It will start emergency medical help on its way as fast as possible. When calling 9-1-1 or the local emergency number, describe the victim's condition to the dispatcher. Do not hang up before the dispatcher does. You might cut off

**If the victim doesn't respond to you in any way, assume the victim is unconscious. Call 9-1-1 or the local emergency number at once!**

# "Do No Further Harm"

One of the most dangerous threats to a seriously injured victim is unnecessary movement. Usually when giving care, you will not face dangers that require you to move a victim. In most cases, you can follow the emergency steps (Check—Call—Care) where you find the victim. Moving the victim can cause additional injury and pain and complicate the victim's recovery.

There are three general situations in which you should move a victim. The most obvious is when you are faced with immediate danger such as fire, lack of oxygen, risk of explosion or a collapsing structure.

A second reason to move a victim is if you have to get to another victim who may have a more serious problem. In this case, you may have to move a victim with minor injuries to reach one who needs care immediately.

Third, you may have to move the victim to provide proper care. For example, someone who has collapsed and does not show signs of circulation needs CPR. CPR needs to be performed on a firm, level surface. If the surface or space is not adequate to provide care, the victim should be moved.

Once you decide to move a victim, you must quickly decide how to move the victim. Carefully consider your safety and the safety of the victim. Base your decision on the dangers you are facing, the size and condition of the victim, your ability and condition and whether you have any help.

You can improve your chances of successfully moving a victim without injuring yourself. When you lift, use your legs, not your back. Bend your body at the knees and hips and avoid twisting your body. Walk forward when possible, taking small steps and looking where you are going.

Avoid twisting or bending the victim with a possible head, neck or back injury. Do not move a victim who is too large to move comfortably.

You can help support a victim who is conscious and who can walk with assistance. Place the victim's arm over your shoulders and hold it in place with your hand. Support the victim with your other arm around the victim's waist. If you have another person to help you, he or she can support the victim the same way on the other side.

If you have a second responder to help, you can also carry a victim who cannot walk. The seat carry provides a secure way for two people to carry a victim. The two responders face each other and interlock their arms, each with one arm under the victim's thighs and one

**The clothes drag.**

arm behind the victim's back. The victim is lifted by the seat formed by the responders' arms.

If you are alone and the victim cannot walk with assistance, you can drag the victim. Use the victim's clothes (e.g., shirt, coat or sweater) to drag the victim if you suspect a head, neck or back injury. Gather the victim's clothes tightly behind the victim's neck. Use the clothes to pull the victim. Support the head with the clothes and your hands.

**The walking assist.**

**The two-person seat carry.**

CALL DIAL 9 1 1

some information the dispatcher needs. Whenever possible, ask a bystander to make the call for you.

If you are the only person on the scene, shout for help. If no help arrives, *Call First,* that is, call 9-1-1 or the local emergency number before providing care for—

- An unconscious adult or child 8 years old or older.
- An unconscious infant or child known to be at high risk for heart problems.

*Call First* situations are likely to be cardiac emergencies, such as sudden cardiac arrest, where the *time factor is critical.* The research shows that the shorter time from collapse to first shock using an automated external defibrillator (AED), the greater the chance of survival for an adult or child 8 years old or older. For an infant or child with a known risk for heart problems, early access to the EMS system and the emergency medical care that results increases the chance of survival.

*Call Fast* situations are likely to be breathing, bleeding and other non-cardiac emergencies. When you are alone in these

types of situations, provide 1 minute of care, then,

*Call Fast* for—

- An unconscious victim less than 8 years old.
- Any victim of submersion or near drowning.
- Any victim of cardiac arrest associated with trauma.
- Any victim of drug overdose.

In *Call Fast* situations, the conditions are often related to breathing emergencies, rather than sudden cardiac arrest. In these situa-

**Calling for help is often the most important step you can take to help the victim.**

tions, provide support for airway, breathing and circulation through rescue breaths or chest compressions as appropriate.

When making the call, find the nearest telephone as quickly as possible. Make the call and go back to the victim. Recheck the victim and give the necessary care. Call 9-1-1 or the local emergency number if the victim is unconscious. You should also call if a victim is faint, drowsy, confused, dizzy or drifts in and out of consciousness.

Call if a victim is having trouble breathing or is breathing in an unnatural way. A victim who is breathing very slowly, heavily or rapidly or gasping for breath might not be getting enough air or may stop breathing. A victim who is making shrill, gurgling or choking noises may be in similar danger.

A victim who shows no signs of circulation may not have a beating heart. Signs of circulation include normal breathing, coughing or movement in response to rescue breaths and a pulse. A victim who is bleeding severely will quickly die after losing a large amount of blood. These are life-threatening conditions requiring the rapid assistance of emergency medical professionals.

Other conditions may be less obvious but no less dangerous. A victim with persistent discomfort, pain or pressure in the chest or abdomen may well have internal injuries you cannot see as may the victim who is vomiting or passing blood.

Multiple seizures, a seizure that lasts longer than 5 minutes, a severe headache and slurred speech can all be signals of serious injury. The victim may be poisoned, have a head, neck or back injury or have some other dangerous condition, so call 9-1-1 or the local emergency number. If you suspect the victim has one or more broken bones, be sure to call 9-1-1 or the local emergency number for help. If not cared for properly, fractures can cause both immediate and long-term problems.

You also need to call 9-1-1 or the local emergency number for certain situations that must be dealt with only by trained and properly equipped people. Fire and explosion are situations of this type and so are downed electrical wires and swiftly moving or rapidly rising water. They make a scene unsafe and you must always stay at a safe distance when any of these conditions are part of any emergency scene.

Poisonous gas can be harder to detect. Sometimes it has no odor or color. You might suspect poisonous gas is present if you see people who are unconscious or behaving strangely for no apparent reason. Call 9-1-1 or the local emergency number. Call also for vehicle collisions and for situations in which victims cannot be reached or moved easily. They may be trapped in cars or in

# When To Call

**EMS**

**If the victim is unconscious, have someone else call 9-1-1 or the local emergency number immediately while you provide care. Use *Call First* and *Call Fast* to help you remember when to make the call in a situation where you are the only responder. Sometimes a conscious victim will tell you not to call an ambulance and you may not be sure what to do. Call 9-1-1 or the local emergency number if the victim—**

- Is or becomes unconscious.
- Has trouble breathing or is breathing in a strange way.
- Has chest discomfort, pain or pressure that persists for more than 3-5 minutes or that goes away and comes back.
- Is bleeding severely.
- Has pressure or pain in the abdomen that does not go away.
- Is vomiting or passing blood.
- Has a seizure that lasts more than 5 minutes or multiple seizures.
- Has a seizure and is pregnant.
- Has a seizure and is diabetic.
- Has a severe headache or slurred speech.
- Appears to have been poisoned.
- Has injuries to the head, neck or back.
- Has possible broken bones.

# Also Call

**Also call for any of these situations:**
- Fire or explosion
- Downed electrical wires
- Swiftly moving or rapidly rising water
- Presence of poisonous gas
- Vehicle collisions
- Victims who cannot be moved easily

# HOW TO

# CALL EMS

*The most important step*

*you can take for a victim*

*who is unconscious or has*

*some other life-threatening*

*condition is to call for emer-*

*gency medical help. Make*

*the call quickly and return*

*to the victim. If possible,*

*send someone else to make*

*the call. Be sure that you or*

*another caller follows these*

*four steps:*

**1** Call the local emergency number. The number is 9-1-1 in many communities. In others, it is a seven- or ten-digit number. Dial 0 (the operator) if you do not know the number in the area.

**2** Give the dispatcher the necessary information. Answer any questions that he or she might ask. Most dispatchers will ask—

- The exact location or address of the emergency. Include the name of the city or town, nearby intersections, nearby landmarks, the building name, the floor and the room or apartment number.
- The caller's name.
- What happened—for example, a motor vehicle collision, fire or fall.
- How many people are involved.
- The condition of the victim(s)—for example, unconsciousness, chest pains or severe bleeding.
- What help (first aid) is being given.

**3** Do not hang up until the dispatcher hangs up. The EMS dispatcher may be able to tell you how best to care for the victim.

**4** Return and continue to care for the victim.

With a life-threatening condition, the survival of a victim often depends on both emergency medical help and the care you can provide. You will have to use your best judgment, based on knowledge of your surroundings, knowledge gained from this course and other training you may have received to make the decision to call. It is often a good idea to ask a bystander to make the call while you provide care.

# WHAT HAPPENS WHEN YOU CALL EMS

When your call is answered, you will be talking to an emergency dispatcher who has had special training in dealing with crises over the phone.

The dispatcher will ask you for your phone number and address and will ask other key questions to determine whether you need police, fire or medical assistance.

It may seem that the dispatcher asks a lot of questions. Focus on remaining calm so that you can give clear answers. The information you give will help the dispatcher to send the type of help you need, based on the severity of the emergency.

Once EMS is on the way, the dispatcher may stay on the line and continue to talk with you. Many dispatchers are also trained to give instructions before EMS arrival, so they can assist you with certain life-saving techniques, such as CPR, rescue breathing or the use of an AED, until EMS arrives.

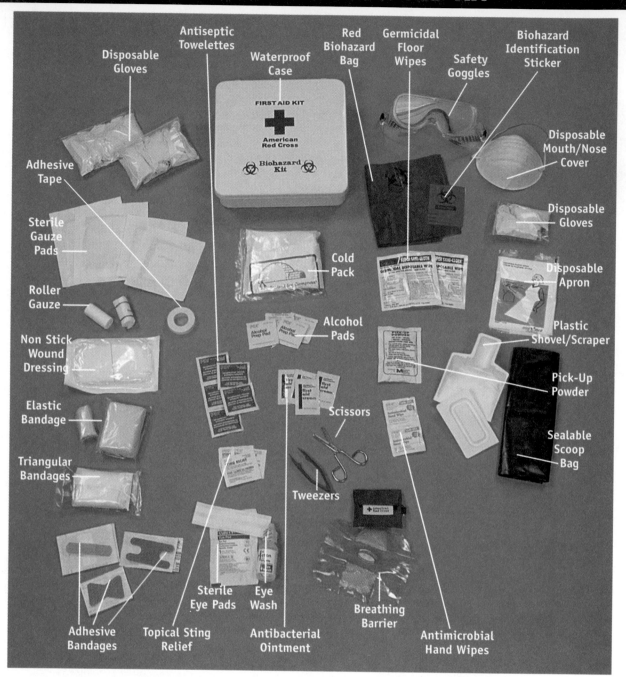

Disposable Gloves

Antiseptic Towelettes

Waterproof Case

Red Biohazard Bag

Germicidal Floor Wipes

Safety Goggles

Biohazard Identification Sticker

FIRST AID KIT

American Red Cross

Biohazard Kit

Disposable Mouth/Nose Cover

Adhesive Tape

Sterile Gauze Pads

Roller Gauze

Non Stick Wound Dressing

Elastic Bandage

Triangular Bandages

Cold Pack

Alcohol Pads

Scissors

Tweezers

Disposable Gloves

Disposable Apron

Plastic Shovel/Scraper

Pick-Up Powder

Sealable Scoop Bag

Adhesive Bandages

Topical Sting Relief

Sterile Eye Pads

Eye Wash

Antibacterial Ointment

Breathing Barrier

Antimicrobial Hand Wipes

A well-stocked first aid kit is a handy thing to have. To be prepared for emergencies, keep a first aid kit in your home and in your automobile. Carry a first aid kit with you or know where you can find one when you are hiking, biking, camping or boating. Find out the location of first aid kits where you work.

First aid kits come in many shapes and sizes. You can buy one from a drug store or your local Red Cross chapter may sell them. You can make your own first aid kit. Some kits are designed for specific activities, such as hiking, camping or boating. Whether you buy a first aid kit or put one together, make sure it has all the items you may need. Include any personal items, such as medications and emergency phone numbers or other items your health-care provider may suggest. Check the kit regularly. Make sure the flashlight batteries work. Check expiration dates and replace any used or out-of-date contents.

buildings, for example. Call also for emergencies involving more than one victim.

These circumstances are not a complete list. There are always exceptions. Trust your instincts. If you think there is an emergency, there probably is. If you are confused or unsure about what care to give, call 9-1-1 or the local emergency number at once. EMS personnel would rather come and find no emergency than arrive at an emergency too late to help.

## CARE

Once you have checked the scene and the victim, you may need to provide care. To do this, you can follow some general steps. Always care for life-threatening emergencies before those that are not life threatening. While waiting for EMS personnel to arrive, watch for changes in the victim's breathing and consciousness. Help the victim rest comfortably. Keep him or her from getting chilled or overheated. Reassure the victim.

If the victim is conscious and able to talk, he or she is breathing and shows signs of circulation. In-troduce yourself and then get permission from the victim so that you can help. Ask what happened and if the victim has pain. Ask where the pain is located and what it is like—burning, aching, sharp, stinging. Ask when it started and how bad it is. Be calm and patient. Speak normally and simply.

Always care for life-threatening emergencies first!

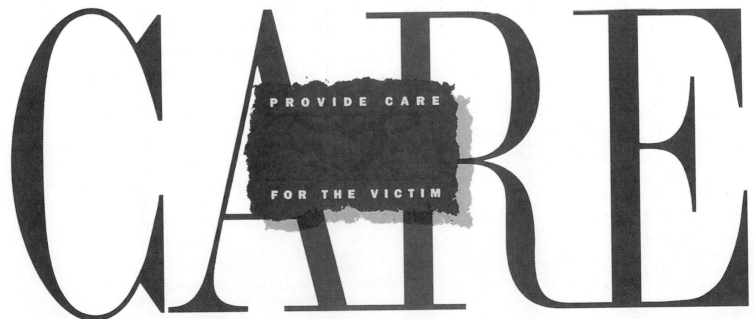

CARE

PROVIDE CARE

FOR THE VICTIM

After you have finished checking the victim and giving care, you might decide to take the victim to a hospital or doctor yourself. **Be very careful about making this decision.** *Do not* transport a victim with a life-threatening condition or one that could become life threatening.

A car trip can be painful for the victim. It can also make an injury worse. If you do decide to transport the victim, always have someone else come with you. Watch the victim carefully for any changes in condition. Be sure you know the fastest route. **Do not let the victim drive, either alone or with you.**

When you respond to an emergency, remember the emergency action steps: Check—Call—Care. They will guide your actions in an emergency and ensure your safety and the safety of others. By following these steps, you can give the victim of a serious illness or injury the best chance of survival.

## Don't Cry Wolf!

Your local emergency number is just for that—emergencies! It should not be misused. Non-emergency calls account for about 30 to 40 percent of all 9-1-1 calls in many U.S. cities. So please, use good judgment.

# DEVELOPING A PLAN OF

# ACTIO

**E**mergencies can happen quickly. There may be no time to think about what you should do. There may be only enough time to react. You can improve your reaction and change the outcome of the emergency by planning.

Everyone has a plan of action. It may be instinct. It may be as simple as, "I'm scared...run!" Running may even work—if you can run fast enough and in the right direction. Most of us do not want to base how well we deal with emergencies on how fast we run. We would rather find a way to improve our chances. We need a well-thought-out plan.

A good plan identifies the emergencies you are most likely to face. The plan also identifies the possible location and the persons involved. All of this information can help you to define the size and scope of a possible emergency. Now, you can begin to decide how you would respond and what you would need.

The first step in planning is to gather information. Here are some suggestions on where to start.

**First, think about your home.**
- Type of home (mobile, high rise duplex, single family, etc.)
- Type of construction (wood, brick, etc.)
- Location of sleeping areas
- Number and location of smoke alarms
- Location of gasoline, solvent or paint storage

- Number and types of locks on doors
- Location of telephones
- Location of flashlights
- Location of fire extinguisher
- Location of first aid kit

**Think about who lives there.**
- Number of people living in the home
- Number of people over 65 or under 6 years of age
- Number of people sleeping above or below the ground floor
- Number of people unable to exit without help

**Think about the types of emergencies that you may face at home.**
- Injuries (like a fall or a cut)
- Illnesses (like a stroke or a heart attack)
- Natural disasters (like a tornado or an earthquake)
- Fire

**Now that you have information, you can start a plan.**
Get help from the people you live with. Write the list of emergencies and under each emergency, list—
1. The way the emergency would affect your home.
2. The way you would like the people in your home to react.
3. The steps you have taken to prevent or minimize the effect of the emergency.
4. The steps you need to take.

**For example, when discussing fire you might list—**
1. The fire could burn all or part of our home.
2. If the fire started on the stove while someone was cooking, that person should use a fire extinguisher to put out the fire. If the fire could not be controlled, he or she should call the emergency number, have everyone leave the house and leave also. Then everyone should meet at the tree in the front yard.
3. Smoke alarms are in the kitchen, the stairwells and outside the bedrooms. A fire extinguisher is in the kitchen.
4. We should make sure the fire extinguisher is charged and everyone should know how to operate it. We should also make sure everyone knows what to do.

**If you need more help, here are other sources of information:**
- Insurance companies
- Your city or county Emergency Management office
- Your police department
- Your fire department/rescue squad

Try to imagine as many situations as possible for each emergency. Think about emergencies away from home. Use the same process to decide what to do. When people have questions, others living in the home can help decide what action to take.

When you reach a decision, write it down. You now have a personal plan. Practice it. Keep it current.

# FIRST AID CHALLENGE

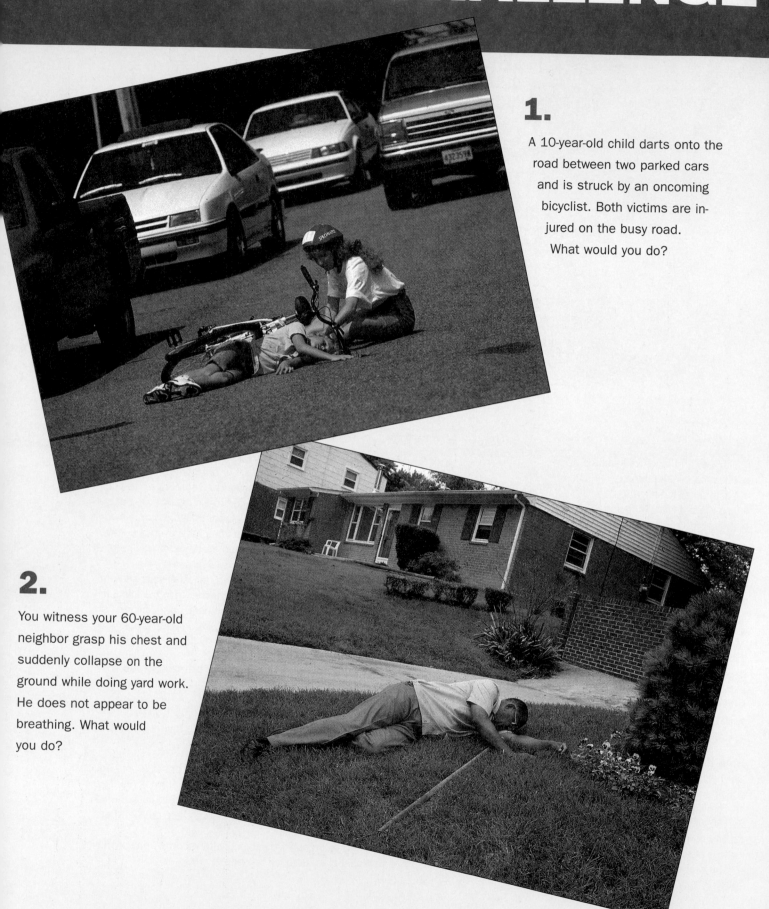

**1.**

A 10-year-old child darts onto the road between two parked cars and is struck by an oncoming bicyclist. Both victims are injured on the busy road. What would you do?

**2.**

You witness your 60-year-old neighbor grasp his chest and suddenly collapse on the ground while doing yard work. He does not appear to be breathing. What would you do?

You have learned the emergency action steps that can be applied in any emergency—check, call, and care. Would you know what to do in an emergency? Test your knowledge of the emergency action steps by deciding what you would do in each of the four situations below. If you are unsure how you should proceed in any of the four situations, review the information in "Taking Action."

## 3.

Your 50-year-old relative has been complaining of an "unusual tightness" in her chest and nausea for several hours. Suddenly she experiences severe pain in her chest and is now having trouble breathing. What would you do?

## 4.

A pitcher on a little league baseball team has been struck in the ankle by a line-drive. He falls to the ground in pain and is unable to move his foot. What would you do?

# CHECKING

When you reach the victim, check first for life-threatening conditions, such as

unconsciousness. In many emergencies, you will know right away whether the

victim is unconscious. However, in some situations,

you may not be able to tell. If you are not sure

whether a victim is unconscious, tap the victim

on the shoulder.

Always begin by determining if a victim is conscious. To find out if a victim is conscious, tap him or her on one shoulder. Ask the victim if he or she is OK. If you know the person, use his or her name. Speak loudly. If the victim does not respond to you, assume he or she is unconscious. Have someone else call 9-1-1 or the local emergency number.

# THE VICTIM

## CHECKING AN UNCONSCIOUS ADULT/CHILD

If you are alone and have to call 9-1-1 or the local emergency number yourself, you should return immediately to the victim. Whenever possible, send another person to make the call while you provide care. You must find out if there are other conditions that threaten the victim's life. You should check to see if an unconscious victim—

- Has an open airway.
- Is breathing.
- Shows signs of circulation.
- Is bleeding severely.

An easy way to recall what you need to check is to remember ABC: Airway (open the airway), Breathing (check for breathing) and Circulation (check for signs of circulation and severe bleeding). If the victim is not breathing, the victim's life is threatened. To check to see if a victim who is unconscious is breathing, put your head near the victim's mouth and nose without moving the victim. Look, listen and feel for breathing for about 5 seconds. If you cannot tell if the victim is breathing, turn the victim to a face-up position. In this case,

**If the victim does not respond to you, assume he or she is unconscious. Call 9-1-1 or the local emergency number at once!**

# Check to see if an unconscious victim—
- **Is Breathing.**
- **Shows Signs of Circulation.**
- **Is Bleeding Severely.**

roll the victim gently onto his or her back. While rolling the victim, be sure to keep the head, neck and back in as straight a line as possible.

Tilt the victim's head back and lift the chin, then recheck breathing for about 5 seconds. If the victim is breathing, the victim's heart is beating and circulating blood. If the victim is not breathing, you must immediately give the victim 2 rescue breaths. Then find out if the victim's heart is beating by checking for signs of circulation, which include normal breathing, coughing or movement in response to rescue breaths and a pulse. Be sure to check for signs of circulation **for no more than 10 seconds.**

To check the pulse in an adult or a child, feel at the front of the neck for the Adam's apple and slide your fingers into the groove next to it in the side of the neck. If the heart is beating, you will feel the beat of the blood in one of the big blood vessels (carotid artery) that runs along both sides of the neck. With an infant, feel for a pulse in either arm midway between the elbow and the shoulder (brachial artery). **Take no more than 10 seconds to check for signs of circulation.**

If the victim shows signs of circulation but is still not breathing, you will have to give rescue breaths. If the victim does not show signs of circulation, the heart is not beating properly. You

**To check for breathing, look, listen and feel for breathing for about 5 seconds. Watch the chest to see if it clearly rises.**

To find out if the heart is beating, check for signs of circulation for no more than 10 seconds. To check for signs of circulation, look for normal breathing, coughing or movement in response to rescue breaths and a pulse. To check for a pulse of an adult or child, feel for one at the side of the neck (in the groove next to the Adam's apple). Check the pulse of an infant at the inside of the arm between the shoulder and the elbow.

**Adult**

**Child**

**Infant**

must keep blood circulating in the victim's body until emergency medical help arrives. To do this, you will have to give cardiopulmonary resuscitation (CPR). Rescue breathing and CPR are discussed in a later section called "When Seconds Count."

Check for bleeding by looking over the victim's body from head to toe for signs of bleeding, such as blood-soaked clothing. Bleeding is severe, for example, when blood spurts out of a wound. Bleeding usually looks worse than it is. A small amount of blood on a slick surface or mixed with water almost always looks like a great deal of blood. It is not always easy to recognize severe bleeding. You will have to make a decision based on your best judgment. If you think bleeding is severe, call 9-1-1 or the local emergency number immediately.

## CHECKING A CONSCIOUS VICTIM

If the victim is conscious, ask what happened. If the victim is able to speak, he or she is breathing and shows signs of circulation. Look for other life-threatening conditions and conditions that might become life threatening.

**Step 1:** **Check the scene for safety, then check the victim...**Tap the victim's shoulder and shout to see if the victim responds.

**If no response...**Call, or have someone else call, 9-1-1 or the local emergency number.

**Step 2:** **Open the airway. Look, listen and feel for breathing for about 5 seconds.**

**If the victim is face-down...**Check for breathing in the position that you find the victim.

**If the victim is face-up...** Open the airway, then check for breathing.

**Step 3:** **If the face-down victim is not breathing or you cannot tell...**Roll the victim onto his or her back while supporting the head, neck and back. Open the airway. Look, listen and feel for breathing for about 5 seconds.

**Step 4:** **If the victim is unconscious but breathing and shows signs of circulation...** Place him or her in a recovery position.

**Step 5:** **If the victim is not breathing or you cannot tell...** Give 2 rescue breaths.

**Step 6:** **If breaths go in... Check for signs of circulation for no more than 10 seconds.** Check for severe bleeding. Give care for the conditions you find.

**If breaths do not go in... GO TO** "Unconscious Choking—Adult," Step 1, Page 76 **OR** "Unconscious Choking—Child," Step 1, Page 110.

# Checking an Unconscious Infant

**Step 1:** **Check the scene for safety, then check the infant...**
Check the infant by flicking the foot or tapping the shoulder and shouting.

**If no response...**
Call, or have someone else call, 9-1-1 or the local emergency number.

**Step 2:** **Open the airway. Look, listen and feel for breathing for about 5 seconds.**

**Step 3:** **If the infant is breathing...Monitor ABCs.**

**Step 4:** **If the infant is NOT breathing or you cannot tell...**Give 2 rescue breaths.

**Step 5:** **If breaths go in...** Check for signs of circulation for no more than 10 seconds. Check for severe bleeding. Give care for the conditions you find.

**If breaths do not go in... GO TO** "Unconscious Choking—Infant," Step 1, Page 127.

**Medical alert tags can provide important medical information about the victim.**

The victim may be able to tell you what happened and how he or she feels. This information helps determine what care may be needed.

This check has three possible steps:

1. Talk to the victim and to any people who saw the emergency take place.
2. Check an adult victim from head to toe so you do not overlook any problems.
3. Check an infant or child from toe to head. This will be less emotionally threatening. For young children, you may find that checking the child while he or she is seated in the parent's or guardian's lap is helpful.

Do not ask the victim to move and do not move the victim yourself.

Check the victim's head by examining the scalp, face, ears, nose and mouth. Look for cuts, bruises, bumps or depressions. Watch for changes in consciousness. Notice if the victim is drowsy, not alert or confused. Look for changes in the victim's breathing. A healthy person breathes normally, quietly and easily. Infants and young children generally breathe faster than adults. Breathing that is not normal includes noisy breathing such as gasping for air; making rasping, gurgling or whistling sounds; breathing unusually fast or slow; and breathing that is painful.

Notice how the skin looks and feels. Note if the skin is reddish, pale or ashen. Feel with the back of your hand on the forehead to see if the skin feels unusually damp, dry, cool or hot. The skin can provide clues that the victim is injured or sick.

Look over the body. Ask again about any areas that hurt. Ask the victim to move each part of the body that does not hurt. Check the shoulders by asking

the victim to shrug them. Check the chest and abdomen by asking the victim to take a deep breath. Ask the victim if he or she can move the fingers, hands and arms. Check the hips and legs in the same way. *During a head-to-toe check, do not touch any painful areas; do not ask the victim to move any parts that hurt.* Watch the victim's face and listen

**If a victim is able to talk, you know he or she is breathing and shows signs of circulation.**

for signals of discomfort or pain as you check for injuries.

Look for odd bumps or depressions. Think of how the body usually looks. If you are not sure a body part or limb appears unusual, check it against the opposite limb or the other side of the body.

Look for a medical alert tag on the victim's wrist, neck or ankle. A tag will give you medical information about the victim, care to give for that problem and who to call for help.

When you have finished checking, if the victim can move his or her body without any pain and there are no other signs of injury, have the victim rest sitting up. When the victim feels ready, help him or her stand up.

As you continue reading you will learn more about life-threatening emergencies, such as breathing and heart problems.

Changing everyday habits can improve the quality of your life and reduce the possibility of illness and injury. The following list of statements can help you to identify some important steps toward a healthier and safer life. Mark each box next to the statement that represents your actions. Unmarked boxes identify areas that put you at risk.

## Stress

- [ ] 1. I plan my days off to allow time for recreation.
- [ ] 2. I get enough sleep.
- [ ] 3. I express feelings of anger and worry.
- [ ] 4. I make decisions with little or no worry.
- [ ] 5. I set realistic goals for myself.
- [ ] 6. I accept responsibility for my actions.
- [ ] 7. I manage stress so that it does not affect my physical well-being.
- [ ] 8. I discuss problems with friends and relatives.

## Physical Health

- [ ] 1. I eat a balanced diet.
- [ ] 2. I have regular medical check-ups.
- [ ] 3. I have regular dental check-ups.
- [ ] 4. I have regular eye examinations.
- [ ] 5. I avoid using illegal substances.
- [ ] 6. I have fewer than five alcoholic beverages per week.
- [ ] 7. I avoid using alcoholic beverages when taking medications.
- [ ] 8. When taking medications, I follow the directions on the label.
- [ ] 9. I avoid tobacco use and exposure to others' smoke.
- [ ] 10. I avoid exposure to sunlight by using protection to prevent skin and eye damage.

## Personal Safety

- [ ] 1. I keep my vehicle in good operating condition.
- [ ] 2. I obey traffic laws.
- [ ] 3. I wear safety belts whenever I operate a motor vehicle or when I ride as a passenger in a motor vehicle.
- [ ] 4. I keep recreational equipment in good working condition.
- [ ] 5. I wear life jackets (personal flotation devices—PFDs) when taking part in water activities, such as boating, fishing and waterskiing.
- [ ] 6. I swim only when others are present.
- [ ] 7. I wear a helmet when using a bicycle, motorcycle, all-terrain vehicle, scooter, skateboard or roller blades.

## Home Safety

- [ ] 1. I post local emergency number(s) near my telephone(s).
- [ ] 2. I have battery-operated smoke alarms where I live.
- [ ] 3. I keep medications safely and securely stored out of the reach of children.
- [ ] 4. I keep cleansers and other poisonous materials safely and securely stored.
- [ ] 5. I turn off the oven and other appliances after use.
- [ ] 6. I keep a working fire extinguisher in my home.
- [ ] 7. I have a carbon monoxide alarm in my home.
- [ ] 8. I have an emergency plan in the event of injury, sudden illness or natural disaster.
- [ ] 9. I practice emergency plans with my family or roommates.

HEALTH CHECK

HEALTHY LIFE-STYLE IQ QUIZ

WHEN

# SECONDS COUNT

## ADULT LIFE-THREATENING EMERGENCIES

In a life-threatening emergency, you must help at once.

It may only be a matter of seconds before the person dies. An emergency is life threatening if the victim is unconscious, is not breathing, has trouble breathing, shows no signs of circulation or is bleeding severely.

Fortunately, most of the victims you encounter will be conscious. Very likely, they will be able to indicate what is wrong by speaking to you or by gesturing. You will be able to ask them questions. But when a person cannot be aroused, it is difficult to know what is wrong, besides being unconscious. Unconsciousness is a life-threatening emergency. You need to have someone call 9-1-1 or the local emergency number while you continue to check the victim to see if he or she is breathing, shows signs of circulation or is bleeding severely.

You may have to care for a person who is unconscious but who is breathing normally and shows signs of circulation. For example, a person might have hit his or her head in a fall or just fainted. In such cases, make sure someone has called 9-1-1 or the local emergency number. There is no need to move the person as long as he or she is breathing normally. If the person vomits, roll him or her onto one side and clear the mouth and throat. If the person stops breathing, place the person on his or her back and breathe for the person as described later in this manual. If you are alone and have to leave the person for any reason, such as to call for help, place the person in the recovery position in case he or she vomits while you are gone.

Once in the recovery position, the victim should be turned to the opposite side after 30 minutes or if there are signs of loss of circulation to the lower arm, such as pale, ashen or grayish skin that is cool to the touch. If there is a suspected head, neck or back injury and a clear, open airway can be maintained, do not move the victim unnecessarily. If a clear airway cannot be maintained, the victim should be moved to his or her side keeping the head, neck or back in a straight line. This position is not recommended for infants because of the risk of Sudden Infant Death Syndrome (SIDS).

Most often, unconsciousness is a signal that a victim may have other life-threatening conditions. A person who is unconscious will soon die if breathing stops and if the heart stops. You must discover and care for these conditions as quickly as possible.

0 minutes: **Breathing stops. Heart will soon stop beating.**

4–6 minutes: **Brain damage possible.**

6–10 minutes: **Brain damage likely.**

Over 10 minutes: **Irreversible brain damage certain.**

**Time is critical in life-threatening emergencies. Unless the brain gets oxygen within minutes of when breathing stops, brain damage or death will occur.**

**If vomiting occurs, roll the victim on the side, and clear the mouth of any matter.**

**Whenever the victim is breathing and unconscious or you are alone and must leave the victim, and you do not suspect a head, neck or back injury, then place the victim in the recovery position in case he or she vomits.**

# OXYGEN IS VITAL TO LIFE

The body requires a constant supply of oxygen to survive. When you breathe air in through the nose and mouth, it travels down the throat, through the windpipe and into the lungs. This path from the nose and mouth to the lungs is called the airway.

When the air you breathe reaches the lungs, oxygen from the air is transferred to the blood and is circulated to all parts of the body through large blood vessels called arteries. Injuries and illnesses that affect breathing or the action of the heart or cause bleeding can interrupt the supply of oxygen. When enough oxygen does not reach the lungs or does not circulate properly in the body, it is a life-threatening condition. You must act immediately.

# SIGNALS

## OF

# BREATHING EMERGENCIES

Breathing is unusually slow or rapid.

Breaths are unusually deep or shallow.

Victim is gasping for breath.

Victim is wheezing, gurgling or making high-pitched noises.

Victim's skin is unusually moist.

Victim's skin has a flushed, pale or ashen appearance.

Victim feels short of breath.

Victim feels dizzy or lightheaded.

Victim feels discomfort or pain in the chest or tingling in hands or feet.

## Breathing Emergencies

The body requires a constant supply of oxygen to survive. When you breathe air through the nose and mouth, it travels down the throat, through the windpipe and into the lungs. The pathway from the nose and mouth to the lungs is commonly called the airway. Once air reaches the lungs, oxygen in the air is transferred to the blood. The blood transports the oxygen to the brain and heart, as well as to all other parts of the body.

Certain emergencies are life threatening because they greatly reduce or eliminate the body's supply of oxygen. For instance, when a person has trouble breathing, that person's body may not get enough oxygen. When breathing stops or when the heart stops, the body gets no oxygen. Unless the brain gets oxygen within a few minutes after breathing stops, brain damage or death will occur.

A breathing problem so severe that it threatens the victim's life is a breathing emergency. In "Checking the Victim," you learned that you have to check to find out whether an unconscious victim is breathing. You also learned that if the victim is breathing, you must determine if he or she is having trouble breathing.

Breathing emergencies can be caused by injury or illness. For example, if the heart stops beating, breathing will stop. Choking and injury or disease in areas of the brain that control breathing can disturb or stop breathing. In an unconscious person, a likely reason for breathing to stop is that the tongue falls back in the throat and blocks the airway.

Damage to the muscles or bones of the chest can make

breathing painful or difficult. Electric shock and drowning can cause breathing to stop. Severe reactions to certain poisons, drugs, insect stings and foods can also cause breathing emergencies. Other causes include anxiety, excitement and conditions such as asthma.

Asthma is a condition that narrows the air passages. This makes breathing difficult, which is frightening. Asthma may be triggered by a reaction to food, pollen, medications, insect stings, chemical irritants or pollutants. Emotional distress or physical activity can also bring on an asthma attack. People with asthma can usually control an attack with medication. They may carry this medication with them.

Asthma is more common in children and young adults than in older people. You can often tell when a person is having an asthma attack by the wheezing noises he or she makes when breathing.

Hyperventilation occurs when a person breathes faster than normal. It often results from fear or anxiety and is most likely to occur in people who are tense and nervous. However, it can also be caused by head injuries, severe bleeding or illnesses, such as high fever, heart failure, lung disease and diabetic emergencies. Asthma

and exercise also can trigger hyperventilation.

People who are hyperventilating have rapid, shallow breathing. They feel as if they cannot get enough air. Often they are afraid and anxious or seem confused. They may say that they feel dizzy or their fingers and toes feel numb and tingly.

Allergic reactions can also cause breathing problems. At first, the reaction may appear only as a rash and a feeling of tightness in the chest and throat, but this condition can become life threatening. The victim's face, neck and tongue may swell, closing the airway.

Severe allergic reactions can be caused by insect stings, certain foods and medications. People who know they have severe allergic reactions to certain things may have learned to avoid them. They may also carry medication to reverse the reaction and may ask you to help them to use it.[7] If not cared for at once, a severe allergic reaction can become life threatening.

Even though there are many causes of breathing problems, you do not need to know the exact cause of a breathing emergency to care for it. You do need

**A person who is having trouble breathing may breathe more easily in a sitting position.**

to be able to recognize when a person is having trouble breathing or is not breathing at all.

## If a Person Has Trouble Breathing

Normal breathing is easy and quiet. The person does not look as if he or she is working hard or struggling to breathe. The person is not making noise when breathing. Breaths are not fast or far apart. Breathing does not cause the person discomfort or pain. The kind of breathing problem you are most likely to encounter

When breathing is too fast, slow, noisy, or painful,

# CALL 9-1-1 OR THE LOCAL EMERGENCY NUMBER
# IMMEDIATELY!

is a conscious person who is having trouble breathing. You can usually identify a breathing problem by watching and listening to the person's breathing and by asking the person how he or she feels. You should also check the victim's skin appearance.

People with breathing problems look as if they cannot catch their breath. They may gasp for air. They may appear to breathe faster or slower than normal. The breaths may be unusually deep or shallow. They may make unusual noises, such as wheezing or gurgling. They may make high-pitched noises in their throats. They may have difficulty talking to you or may not be able to talk at all. Their skin, at first, may be damp and look flushed. Later, it may look pale or ashen because their blood is getting low amounts of oxygen.

People with breathing problems may say they feel dizzy or lightheaded. They may feel discomfort or pain in the chest or tingling in the hands and feet. They may be afraid or anxious.

Recognizing the signals of breathing problems and giving care are often the keys to preventing these problems from becoming more serious emergencies. A breathing problem such as choking can cause the victim to stop breathing entirely. Trouble breathing can be the first signal of a more serious emergency, such as a heart problem.

If a person is having trouble breathing, help him or her rest in a comfortable position.

Usually, sitting is more comfortable than lying down because breathing is easier in that position. If the victim is conscious, check for other conditions. Remember that a person having

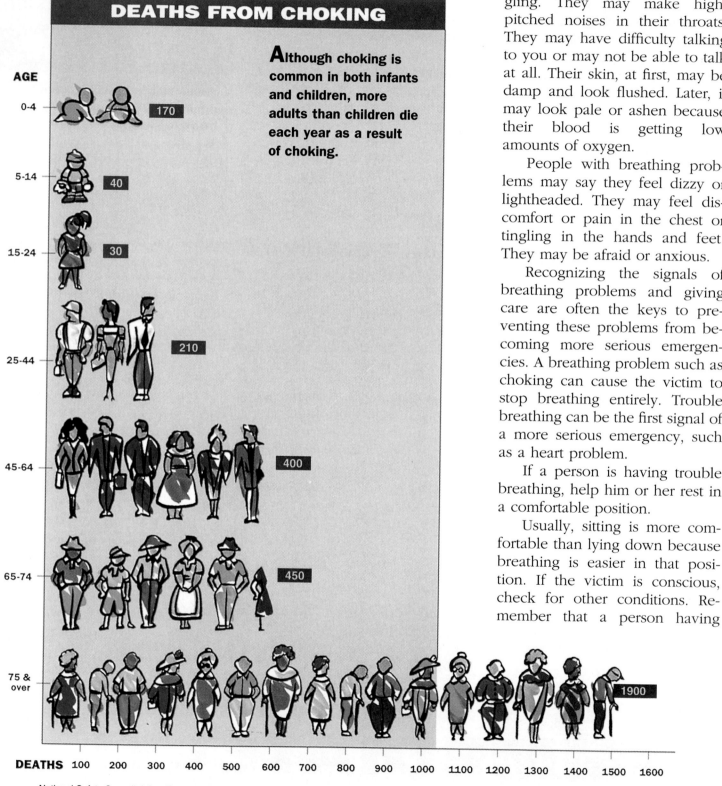

**DEATHS FROM CHOKING**

**A**lthough choking is common in both infants and children, more adults than children die each year as a result of choking.

| AGE | DEATHS |
| --- | --- |
| 0-4 | 170 |
| 5-14 | 40 |
| 15-24 | 30 |
| 25-44 | 210 |
| 45-64 | 400 |
| 65-74 | 450 |
| 75 & over | 1900 |

DEATHS 100 200 300 400 500 600 700 800 900 1000 1100 1200 1300 1400 1500 1600

National Safety Council, Injury Facts, 2000 Edition.

Trying to swallow large pieces of poorly chewed food.

Drinking alcohol before or during meals. (Alcohol dulls the nerves that aid swallowing.)

# Common Causes of Choking

Wearing dentures. (Dentures make it difficult to sense whether food is fully chewed before it is swallowed.)

Eating while talking excitedly, laughing or eating too fast.

Walking, playing or running with food or objects in mouth.

breathing problems may find it hard to talk. Ask bystanders if they know about the victim's condition. The victim can nod or shake his or her head to answer yes-or-no questions. Try to reassure the victim and reduce anxiety. This may make his or her breathing easier.

If the victim is hyperventilating and you are sure it is caused by emotion, such as excitement or fear, tell the victim to relax and breathe slowly. A victim who is hyperventilating from emotion may resume normal breathing if he or she is reassured and calmed down. If the victim's breathing still does not slow down, the victim could have a serious problem.

When breathing is too fast, slow, noisy or painful, call 9-1-1 or your local emergency number immediately.

## If a Conscious Person Is Choking

Choking is a common breathing emergency. A conscious person who is choking has the airway blocked by a piece of food or another object. The airway may be partially or completely blocked. A person whose airway

**Clutching the throat with one or both hands is universally recognized as a distress signal for choking.**

**If a choking person is coughing forcefully, encourage him or her to continue coughing.**

Community First Aid and Safety    **45**

A person who cannot cough forcefully, speak or breathe is choking. Give quick upward thrusts to the abdomen, just above the belly button, until the airway is cleared *(top)*. Give chest thrusts when a choking victim is too big for you to reach around or if the victim is noticeably pregnant.

To give yourself abdominal thrusts, press your abdomen onto a firm object, such as the back of a chair.

is completely blocked cannot breathe at all. With a partially blocked airway, the victim is often still able to breathe, although breathing is difficult.

A person with a partially blocked airway may be able to get enough air in and out of the lungs to cough or to make wheezing sounds. The person may also get enough air to speak. If the choking person is coughing forcefully, let him or her try to cough up the object. A person who is getting enough air to cough or speak is getting enough air to breathe. Stay with the person and encourage him or her to continue coughing. However, if the person continues to cough without coughing up the object, call 9-1-1 or the local emergency number.

A partially blocked airway can very quickly become completely blocked. A person whose airway is completely blocked cannot speak, cough forcefully or breathe. Sometimes the person may cough weakly or make high-pitched noises. This tells you the person is not getting enough air to stay alive. Act at once! Have a bystander call 9-1-1 or the local emergency number while you begin to give care.

When someone is choking, you must get the airway open quickly. To do this, give a series of quick, hard thrusts to the victim's abdomen. These upward thrusts push the abdomen in, putting pressure on the lungs and airway. This forces the air in the lungs to push the object out of the airway—like the cork from a bottle of champagne.

To give abdominal thrusts, stand behind the victim. Wrap your arms around the victim's waist. Make a fist with one hand

SKILL SHEET

If Person is Unable to Speak, Cough, or Breathe...

# Conscious Choking—Adult

**Step 1:** **Check the scene and the victim…**Ask the victim if he or she is choking. Identify yourself and ask the victim if you can help. If the victim is coughing forcefully, encourage continued coughing.

**Step 2:** **If the victim cannot cough, speak or breathe…**
Have someone else call 9-1-1 or the local emergency number.

**Step 3:** **Give abdominal thrusts…**
Stand behind the victim. Place the thumb side of your fist against the middle of the victim's abdomen. Grasp your fist with your other hand and give quick, upward thrusts.

**If the victim becomes unconscious, call 9-1-1, or the local emergency number, if not already done…**
GO TO "Unconscious Choking—Adult," Step 3, Page 76.

and place the thumb side against the middle of the victim's abdomen just above the belly button but below the rib cage. Grab your fist with your other hand and give quick, inward and upward thrusts into the abdomen. Repeat these thrusts until the object is forced out or the victim becomes unconscious. If the victim becomes unconscious, follow the procedures for checking an unconscious choking victim.

If a conscious choking victim is too big for you to reach around and give effective abdominal thrusts, give chest thrusts, such as for a large or obviously pregnant victim. Chest thrusts for a conscious victim are like abdominal thrusts, except for the placement of your hands. Place your fist against the center of the victim's breastbone. Grab it with your other hand and give quick thrusts into the chest.

If you are alone and choking, lean over and press your abdomen against any firm object such as the back of a chair, a railing or the kitchen sink. Do not lean over anything with a sharp edge or corner that might hurt you and be careful when leaning on a rail that is elevated.

## If a Person Is Not Breathing

When a person stops breathing, you have to breathe for that person. This is called rescue

**To give rescue breathing, tilt the head back, lift the chin and pinch the nose shut. Take a breath and breathe slowly into the victim's mouth.**

When a person stops breathing, you have to breathe for that person. This is called

# RESCUE BREATHING

# WHEN YOU GIVE RESCUE BREATHING,

breathe *slowly* into the victim, only until the chest gently rises.

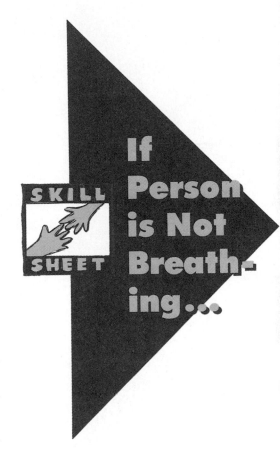

**SKILL SHEET**

**If Person is Not Breathing...**

breathing. It is a way of breathing air into a person that supplies him or her with the oxygen needed to stay alive. Rescue breathing is given to anyone who is unconscious and not breathing but shows signs of circulation.

To give rescue breathing, begin by tilting the head back and lifting the chin to move the tongue away from the back of the throat. This opens the airway, the path that air travels from the nose and mouth to the lungs. Place your ear next to the victim's mouth. Check for breathing by looking at the chest and listening and feeling for breathing for about 5 seconds. If you cannot see, hear or feel any signs of breathing, begin breathing for the victim.

Pinch the victim's nose shut and after taking a breath, make a tight seal around the victim's mouth with your mouth. Breathe slowly and gently into the victim until you see the chest clearly rise. Give 2 rescue breaths, each lasting about 2 seconds for an adult. Pause between rescue breaths to let the air flow out. Watch the victim's chest clearly

rise each time you give a rescue breath to make sure your breaths are going in.

If, any time during your care, you do not see the victim's chest clearly rise as you give rescue breaths, you might not have tilted the head far enough back. Reposition the victim's airway and repeat the breaths. If your breaths still do not go in, the airway is probably blocked. The airway can become blocked by the tongue falling back in the throat, by food, by an object such as a coin or by fluids such as blood or saliva. You will learn how to clear a blocked airway in a later lesson ("If Air Does Not Go In").

Check for signs of circulation after giving these 2 initial rescue breaths. Signs of circulation include normal breathing, coughing or movement in response to rescue breaths and a pulse. In an adult, check for a pulse by finding the Adam's apple and sliding your fingers toward you and down into the groove at the side of the victim's neck. Be sure to check for signs of circulation and breathing **for no more than 10 seconds.**

If there are signs of circulation

# Rescue Breathing—Adult

*Complete "Checking an Unconscious Adult/Child," Pages 32-33.*

**Step 1:** **If the victim shows signs of circulation but is NOT breathing...**Keep the airway open. Seal your mouth tightly around the victim's mouth and pinch the nose shut. Give 1 rescue breath about every 5 seconds. **Do this for about 1 minute (12 breaths).**

**Step 2:** Recheck for signs of circulation and breathing about every minute.

**If there are no signs of circulation...**
**GO TO** "CPR—Adult," Step 1, Pages 68-69.

**A face shield *(top)* or resuscitation mask *(bottom)*, when placed between your mouth and nose and the victim's, can help prevent you from contacting a person's saliva or other body fluids.**

but the victim is still not breathing, give one rescue breath about every 5 seconds. You can time the rescue breaths by counting out loud, such as: "one one-thousand, two one-thousand, three one-thousand" to keep an even pace. Then take a breath on "four one-thousand" and breathe into the victim on "five one-thousand." Counting this way ensures that you give 1 breath about every 5 seconds. After about 1 minute (12 breaths), recheck for signs of circulation and breathing to make sure the heart is still beating. Recheck for signs of circulation and breathing **for no more than 10 seconds.** If there are signs of circulation but no breathing, continue rescue breathing. Recheck for signs of circulation about every minute (12 breaths). Continue rescue breathing until one of the following happens:

- The scene becomes unsafe.
- The victim begins to breathe on his or her own.
- You are too exhausted to continue.
- Another trained responder takes over for you.

You might not feel comfortable with the thought of giving rescue breathing, especially to someone you do not know. Disease transmission is an understandable worry, even though the chances of getting a disease from giving rescue breaths are extremely low.

Barriers, such as face shields and resuscitation masks you put between your mouth and nose and the victim's, can help protect you from blood and other body fluids, such as saliva. The devices with one-way valves help protect you from breathing the air the victim exhales. If available, face shields can be used instead of direct mouth-to-mouth contact. Some devices are small enough to fit in your pocket or in the glove compartment of your car. You can also keep one in your first aid kit. **Do not** delay rescue breathing while searching for a breathing barrier or learning how to use one.

When you are giving rescue breaths, you want to avoid getting air in the victim's stomach instead of the lungs. This may happen if you breathe too long, breathe too hard or do not open the airway far enough.

To avoid getting air into the victim's stomach, keep the victim's head tilted back. Take a breath first and then breathe *slowly* into the victim, just enough to make the chest clearly rise. Each rescue breath should last about 2 seconds. Pause between breaths long enough for the air in the victim to come out and for you to take another breath.

Air in the stomach can make the victim vomit and cause complications. When an unconscious victim vomits, the contents of the stomach can get into the lungs and block breathing. Air in the stomach also makes it harder for the diaphragm, the large muscle that controls breathing, to move. This makes it harder for the lungs to fill with air.

Even when you are giving rescue breaths properly, the victim may vomit. If this happens, roll the victim onto one side and wipe the mouth clean. If possible, use a protective barrier, such as latex gloves, gauze or even a handkerchief, when cleaning out the mouth. Then roll the victim on his or her back again and continue with rescue breathing if

necessary.

Sometimes you may not be able to make a tight enough seal over the victim's mouth. If you cannot make a tight seal, you can breathe into the nose. With the head tilted back, close the mouth by pushing on the chin. Seal your mouth around the victim's nose and breathe into the nose. If possible, open the victim's mouth between rescue breaths to let the air out.

On rare occasions, you may see an opening in a victim's neck as you tilt the head back to check for breathing. This victim may have had an operation to remove part of the windpipe. The victim breathes through this opening, which is called a stoma, instead of through the mouth or nose. This victim will probably also have some medical alert identification, such as a bracelet, necklace or anklet, identifying this condition. Look, listen and feel for breathing with your ear over the stoma. To give rescue breathing to this victim, breathe into the stoma at the same rate

**To give mouth-to-nose breathing, keep the head tilted back, close the victim's mouth and seal your mouth around the victim's nose. Breathe into the nose.**

You may need to perform rescue breathing on a victim with a stoma, an opening in the front of the neck *(top)*. To check for breathing, look, listen and feel for breaths with your ear over the stoma *(middle)*. To give rescue breathing, seal your mouth around the stoma and breathe into the victim *(bottom)*.

as you would breathe into the mouth.

You should provide 1 minute of care *(Call Fast)* for an unconscious person who has nearly drowned. Get help from trained assistance in getting the person out of the water as quickly and safely as possible. If the victim is not breathing, you will have to breathe for him or her.[8]

Finally, be especially careful when a victim may have a head, neck or back injury. These kinds of injuries can result from a fall from a height greater than the victim's, an automobile collision or a diving mishap. If you suspect such an injury, try not to move the victim's head, neck and back.

The *jaw-thrust maneuver* is a method to open the airway of a victim who may have a head, neck or back injury without tilting the head back. For the jaw-thrust maneuver, place one hand on each side of the victim's head, resting your elbows on the surface on which the victim is lying. Grasp the angles of the victim's lower jaw and lift with both hands. If the lips close, you can pull back on the lower lip with your thumb. Close the victim's nostrils during rescue breathing by placing your cheek tightly against them. Remember that the nonbreathing victim's greatest need is for air. If a person's breathing stops or is restricted long enough, he or she will become unconscious and the heart will stop beating. Blood and oxygen will no longer circulate throughout the body. Other body systems will quickly fail.

**If you suspect a head, neck or back injury, try to open the airway by using the jaw-thrust maneuver.**

It is estimated that 61 million Americans suffer from some form of cardiovascular disease. Nearly 1 million deaths each year are attributed to cardiovascular disease. Of these, more than half result from heart attacks. The good news is that the death rate for heart attacks dropped by about 26 percent and the death rate from stroke dropped about 15 percent between 1988 and 1998.[9] The bad news is that heart attacks are occurring more frequently in those under the age of 40 than a decade ago.[10] Many Americans have shown that they can make many heart-healthy changes in their lives, but there is still room for improvement, especially for young adults and teens who are smoking and overweight in greater numbers than ever before. It is estimated that changes, including stopping smoking, eating right and getting regular exercise, have saved as many as 250,000 lives each year.

For current information about heart attack and coronary heart disease prevention, contact the National Heart, Lung and Blood Institute at http://www.nhlbi.nih.gov

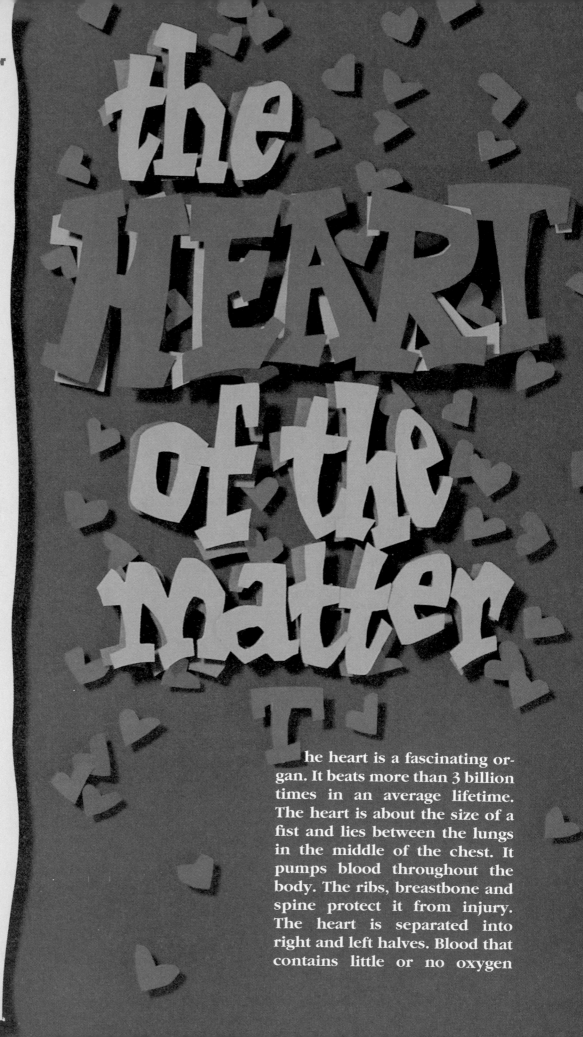

# the HEART of the matter

The heart is a fascinating organ. It beats more than 3 billion times in an average lifetime. The heart is about the size of a fist and lies between the lungs in the middle of the chest. It pumps blood throughout the body. The ribs, breastbone and spine protect it from injury. The heart is separated into right and left halves. Blood that contains little or no oxygen

enters the right side of the heart and is pumped to the lungs. The blood picks up oxygen in the lungs when you breathe. The oxygen-rich blood then goes to the left side of the heart and is pumped to all parts of the body.

The heart needs a constant supply of oxygen. Blood vessels called arteries supply the heart with oxygen-rich blood. Coronary heart disease occurs when fatty deposits containing cholesterol clog the arteries supplying the heart. The arteries become less flexible and are not able to supply blood to the heart. If the heart does not get its blood, it will not work properly. When the heart is behaving normally, it beats evenly and easily, with a steady rhythm. When damage to the heart causes it to stop working effectively, a person experiences

a heart attack. A heart attack can cause the heart to beat in an irregular way. This may prevent blood from circulating effectively. When the heart does not work properly, normal breathing can be disrupted or stopped. A heart attack can also cause the heart to stop beating entirely. This condition is called cardiac arrest.

Any chest pain that is severe, lasts longer than 3-5 minutes, or persists even during rest requires immediate medical care.

## Signals of Heart Problems

A heart attack has some common signals. You should be able to recognize these signals so that you can provide proper care.

The major signal is persistent discomfort, pressure or pain in the chest that does not go away. Unfortunately, it is not always easy to tell heart attack pain from the pain of indigestion, muscle spasms or other conditions. This often causes people to delay obtaining medical care. Brief, stabbing pain or pain that gets worse when you bend or breathe deep is not usually caused by a heart problem.

The pain associated with a heart attack can range from discomfort to an unbearable crushing sensation in the chest. The victim may describe it as pressure, squeezing, tightness, aching or heaviness in the chest. Many heart attacks start slowly, as mild pain or discomfort. Often the victim feels discomfort or pain in the center of the chest. It may spread to the shoulder, arm, neck, jaw or back. The discomfort or pain becomes constant. It is usually not relieved by resting, changing position or taking medicine. Any chest pain that is severe, lasts longer

**The right side receives oxygen-poor blood (blue) from the body and sends it to the lungs where it picks up oxygen. The left side receives oxygen-rich blood (red) from the lungs and pumps it out through the body. One-way valves direct the flow of blood through the heart.**

To upper body

From upper body

Aorta

To lung

To lung

From lung

From lung

**Right Atrium**

**Left Atrium**

**Right Ventricle**

**Left Ventricle**

From lower body

To lower body

Heart attack pain or pressure is often felt in the center of the chest, behind the breastbone. It may spread to the shoulder, neck, arm or jaw.

than 3 to 5 minutes, goes away and comes back or persists even during rest requires medical care at once. Even people who have had a heart attack may not recognize the signals, because the next heart attack(s) can have entirely different signals.

Another signal of a heart attack is trouble breathing. The victim may be breathing faster than normal because the body tries to get much-needed oxygen to the heart. The victim's skin may be pale or ashen, especially around the face. The face may also be damp with sweat. Some heart attack victims sweat heavily or feel dizzy. These signals are caused by the stress put on the body when the heart does not work as it should.

Some people with coronary heart disease may have chest pain or pressure that comes and goes. This type of pain is called angina pectoris, a medical term for pain in the chest. It develops when the heart needs more oxygen than it gets because the arteries leading to the heart are too narrow. When a person with angina is exercising, excited or emotionally upset, the heart might not get enough oxygen. This lack of oxygen can cause chest discomfort or pain.

### Persistent chest discomfort

Victim has persistent chest discomfort, pain or pressure lasting more than 3-5 minutes or that goes away and comes back. Discomfort may range from mild discomfort to an unbearable crushing sensation.

### Discomfort, pain or pressure in either arm; discomfort, pain or pressure that spreads to the shoulder, arm, neck or jaw

### Dizziness or unconsciousness

### Trouble breathing

Victim's breathing is noisy. Victim feels short of breath. Victim breathes faster than normal.

### Nausea

### Skin appearance

Victim's skin may be pale or ashen in color.

### Sweating

Victim's face may be moist or victim may sweat profusely.

The absence of a pulse is the main signal of a cardiac arrest.

## Care for a Heart Attack

**Recognize the signals of a heart attack.**

**Call 9-1-1 or the local emergency number immediately for help.**

**Convince the victim to stop activity and rest.**

**Try to obtain additional information about victim's condition.**

**Comfort the victim.**

**Assist with medication, if prescribed.**

**Monitor the victim's condition.**

**Be prepared to give CPR and to use an AED.**

A person who knows he or she has angina may tell you so. Individuals with angina usually have medicine to take to stop the pain. Stopping physical activity or easing the distress and taking the medicine usually stops the discomfort or pain of angina.

It is important to recognize the signals of a heart attack and act on those signals. Any heart attack may lead to cardiac arrest. Prompt action may prevent it. A heart attack victim whose heart is still beating has a far better chance of living than one whose heart has stopped. Most people who die of a heart attack die within 2 hours after the first signals appear. Many could have been saved if people on the scene or the victim had been aware of the signals and acted promptly. Early treatment with certain medications, for example, can help minimize damage to the heart after a heart attack. To be most effective, these medications need to be given **within 1 hour** of the start of heart attack signals.

Women, the elderly or diabetics may experience signals of a heart attack that are more difficult to recognize. For example, they may experience pain that begins somewhere other than the chest, such as the back, neck or jaw. Also, they may not describe pain, but complain of overall weakness, vague discomfort or a dull aching sensation.[11]

Many heart attack victims delay getting care. Nearly half of them wait for 2 hours or more before going to the hospital.[12] Often they do not realize they are having a heart attack. They may say the signals are just muscle soreness, indigestion or heartburn.

Remember, the key signal of a heart attack is chest discomfort or pain that does not go away. If the pain is severe, does not go away in 3-5 minutes or goes away and comes back, call 9-1-1 or the local emergency number at once. A heart attack victim will probably deny that any signal is serious. Do not let this influence you. If you think the victim might be having a heart attack, act quickly. Call 9-1-1 or the local emergency number.

**Have victim with severe chest pain stop and rest. Many victims find it easier to breathe while sitting.**

## In Case of a Heart Attack

Whenever you suspect that a person is having a heart attack, have the victim stop whatever he or she is doing and rest. Many heart attack victims find it easier to breathe while sitting. If the victim is having persistent chest pain, ask the victim when the discomfort or pain started. Ask what brought the pain on, if anything lessens it, what it feels like and where it hurts. Talk to bystanders and the victim, if possible, to learn more.

Ask the victim if he or she has a history of heart disease. Some people with heart disease have medicine to take for it. You can help by getting the medicine for the victim. If you still think the victim may be having a heart attack or if you are not sure, call 9-1-1 or the local emergency number. Have a bystander call or make the call yourself if you are alone before the victim gets worse and the heart stops. If you think you are having a heart attack, never drive yourself to the hospital.

Be calm and reassuring when caring for a heart attack victim. When you comfort the victim, it helps make him or her less anxious and more comfortable. Watch carefully for any changes in the way the victim looks and behaves. Since the victim may go into cardiac arrest, be prepared to give CPR.

## When the Heart Stops Beating

Cardiac arrest is the condition when the heart stops beating or beats too poorly to circulate blood properly. When cardiac arrest happens, breathing will stop. Cardiac arrest is life threatening. Every year, more than 220,000 victims die of coronary heart disease before they reach a hospital—more than 600 Americans each day.[13]

Heart disease is the most common cause of cardiac arrest. Other causes include drowning, choking, certain drugs, severe injury, brain damage and severe electric shock. These causes can make the heart stop. Cardiac arrest can happen suddenly, without the signals usually seen in a heart attack.

A person in cardiac arrest is unconscious, is not breathing and shows no signs of circulation. The absence of signs of circulation is the main signal of cardiac arrest. No signs of circulation means no blood is going to the brain. Since blood carries oxygen, no oxygen is being supplied to the brain; therefore the brain will die in a few minutes.

Even though a victim is not breathing and shows no signs of circulation, the cells of the brain and of other important organs continue to live for a short time—until all the oxygen in the blood is used. Such a victim needs CPR and probably early defibrillation at once. CPR is a combination of chest compressions and rescue

# A Matter of Choice

Your 75-year-old grandfather is living with your family. He has a terminal illness and is frequently in the hospital. He has no hope of regaining his health.

One afternoon, you go to his room to give him lunch. As you start to talk to him, you realize he has stopped breathing. You check for signs of circulation. He has none. You are suddenly faced with the fact that your grandfather is no longer alive…he's dead. You ask yourself…What do I do?

No one can tell you what to do. No one can advise you. No one can predict the outcome. The decision to try to help your grandfather by giving CPR is a personal one that you must make.

Your mind tells you to give CPR, yet your heart tells you not to. Various questions race through your mind. Can I face the fact I am losing someone I love? Shouldn't I always try to give CPR? What would his life be like after resuscitation? What would grandfather want?

It is important to realize that it is okay to withhold CPR when a terminally ill person is dying. Nature takes its course and in

some cases, people feel they have lived full lives and are prepared for death. Talking to your grandfather about his preferences before such decisions need to be made can help prepare both you and him.

How would this situation have changed if your family and grandfather had planned for this possibility? For instance, what would have happened if your grandfather had planned or given instructions in advance?

Instructions that describe a person's wishes about medical treatment are called advance directives. These instructions make known the person's intentions while he or she is competent to do so and are used when the person can no longer make his or her own health-care decisions.

As provided by the Federal Patient Self-Determination Act, adults who are admitted to a hospital or a health-care facility or who receive assistance from certain organizations that receive funds from Medicare and Medicaid have the right to make fundamental choices about their own care. They must be told about their right to breathing. As you read earlier, rescue breathing supplies oxygen. The presence of signs of circulation means that the heart is circulating this oxygen to the body through the blood. When the heart is not beating, chest compressions are needed to circulate the oxygen. Given together, rescue breathing and chest compressions take over for the heart and lungs. CPR increases a cardiac arrest victim's chances of survival by keeping the brain supplied with oxygen until the victim can receive defibrillation and emergency medical care. Without early CPR and early defibrillation, the brain begins to die in as little as 4 minutes.

make decisions about the level of life support that would be provided in an emergency situation. They would be offered the opportunity to make these choices at the time of admission.

Verbal conversations with relatives, friends or physicians, while the patient is still capable of making decisions, are the most common form of advance directives. However, because conversations may not be recalled accurately or may not have taken into account the illness or emergency now facing the patient, the courts consider written directives more trustworthy.

Two examples of written advance directives are living wills and durable powers of attorney for heath care. The types of health-care decisions covered by these documents vary depending on where you live. Talking with a legal professional can help determine which advance directive options are available in your state and what they do and do not cover.

If your grandfather had established a living will, directions for health care would be in place before he became unable to communicate his wishes. The instructions that can be included in this document vary from state to state. A living will generally allows a person to refuse only medical care that "merely prolongs the process of dying," such as resuscitating a person with a terminal illness.

If your grandfather has established a durable power of attorney for health care, the document would authorize someone to make medical decisions for him in any situation in which he could no longer make them for himself. This authorized person is called a *health-care surrogate* or *proxy*. This surrogate, with the information given by the patient's physician, may consent to or refuse medical treatment on the patient's behalf. In this case, he or she would support the needs and wishes that affect the health-care decisions and the advance directives of your grandfather.

A doctor could formalize your grandfather's preferences by writing "Do Not Resuscitate" (DNR) orders in your

grandfather's medical records. Such orders would state that if your grandfather's heartbeat or breathing stops, he should not be resuscitated. The choice in deciding on DNR orders may be covered in a living will or in the durable power of attorney for health care.

Appointing someone to act as a health-care surrogate, along with writing down your instructions, is the best way to formalize your wishes about medical care.

Some of these documents can be obtained through a personal physician, attorney or various state and health-care organizations. A lawyer is not always needed to execute advance directives. However, if you have any questions concerning advance directives, it is wise to obtain legal advice.

Copies of advance directives should be provided to all personal physicians, family members and the person chosen as the health-care surrogate. Tell them what documents have been prepared and where the original and other copies are located. Discuss the

document with all parties so that they understand the intent of all requests. Keep these documents updated.

Keep in mind that advance directives are not limited to elderly people or people with terminal illnesses. Advance directives should be considered by anyone who has decided on the care he or she would like to have provided. An unexpected illness or injury could create a need for decisions at any time.

Knowing about living wills, durable powers of attorney for health care and DNR orders can help you prepare for difficult decisions. If you are interested in learning more about your rights and the options available to you in your state, contact a legal professional.

REFERENCES
1. Hospital Shared Services of Colorado, Stockard Inventory Program. *Your Right to Make Health Care Decisions.* Denver, Colorado, 1991.
2. Title 42 United States Code Section 1395 cc (a)(1)(Q)(A). Patient Self-Determination Act.

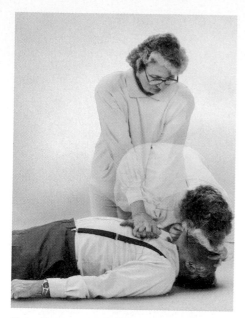

If a victim is not breathing and shows no signs of circulation, he or she needs CPR. CPR is a combination of chest compressions and rescue breathing.

## Cardiac Chain of Survival

CPR provides only about one third the normal blood flow to the brain. CPR alone is not enough to help someone survive cardiac arrest. Emergency medical care is needed as soon as possible. This is why it is so important to call 9-1-1 or the local emergency number immediately. The greatest chance of survival from cardiac arrest occurs when the following sequence of events happens as rapidly as possible:

1. **Early recognition and early access.** The sooner 9-1-1 or the local emergency number is called, the sooner early advanced life support arrives.
2. **Early CPR.** Early CPR helps circulate blood that contains oxygen to the vital organs until an AED is ready to use or emergency medical personnel arrive.
3. **Early defibrillation.** Most victims of sudden cardiac arrest need an electric shock called

# The Shock of Your Life

Every year, about 220,000 Americans collapse and die in their homes, in workplaces or on the streets from coronary heart disease without being hospitalized.[15] Most of these deaths are the result of sudden cardiac arrest. In two thirds of all cardiac arrests the heartbeat flutters wildly before it stops. The electric signals that tell the heart muscle to beat, stop making sense. The heart is unable to send enough blood through the body. This condition is called ventricular fibrillation and can only be

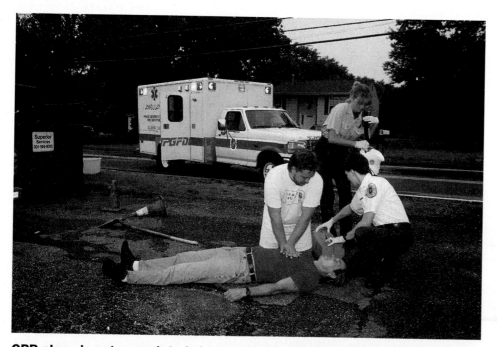

CPR alone is not enough to help someone survive cardiac arrest. Early defibrillation and advanced medical care is needed as soon as possible.

corrected by an electric shock. A heart attack can progress to cardiac arrest or sudden cardiac arrest can happen without warning signals. A victim in cardiac arrest will be unconscious and show no signs of circulation.

Devices that could shock the heart into pumping effectively began to appear in 1966. These devices, called defibrillators, allowed medical personnel, away from the hospital, to monitor the heart's electrical activity. A doctor attached electrodes to the victim's chest to determine the heart's rhythm. If necessary, medical personnel delivered an electric shock to the heart to try to restore the heart's proper rhythm. In addition to doctors, nurses and paramedics eventually began to evaluate rhythms and deliver shocks at the emergency scene. Because of the expense and the lack of trained personnel across the United States, victims were not always able to get the lifesaving help as quickly as they needed.

Today new, easy-to-use automated external defibrillators (AEDs) allow emergency personnel and trained lay responders to provide these lifesaving shocks. The new defibrillators use a computer chip, rather than relying on a medical professional, to analyze the heart's rhythm and deliver a shock if necessary. Typically, the user places two electrode pads on the victim's chest and follows the machine prompts.

Most first responders, like fire fighters and police officers, are trained to use AEDs. By training first responders, communities increase the number of emergency personnel trained to use AEDs. The use of AEDs has been shown to improve survival rates for cardiac arrest in communities adopting widespread defibrillator training for both lay and first responders. Use of CPR and defibrillation within 4 minutes of a sudden cardiac arrest, linked with advanced life support within 8 minutes, almost doubles a victim's chance of survival.

All 50 states recognize and support AED training for lay responders. Authorities are also placing AEDs in areas where large groups of people gather, such as at airports, convention centers, stadiums, large office sites and industrial complexes. Many experts hope that AEDs will soon be as commonplace as fire extinguishers. Contact your local American Red Cross chapter to find out more about AED training.

To give CPR, position yourself so that you can give rescue breaths and chest compressions without having to move.

defibrillation. Each minute that defibrillation is delayed reduces the chance of survival by about 10 percent.

4. **Early advanced life support.** This is given by trained medical personnel who provide further care and transport to hospital facilities.

The above sequence is called the Cardiac Chain of Survival[14]; each link of the chain depends on and is connected to the other links.

As the first step in the Cardiac Chain of Survival, early recognition of a heart attack is critical. Signals of a heart attack include—

- Persistent chest discomfort or pain lasting more than 3-5 minutes or that goes away and comes back.
- Discomfort, pain or pressure in either arm; discomfort, pain or pressure that spreads to the shoulder, arm, neck or jaw.
- Shortness of breath or trouble breathing.
- Nausea.
- Changes in skin appearance.
- Sweating.
- Dizziness or unconsciousness.

It is very important to start CPR promptly and continue it until an AED is available or EMS personnel arrive. Any delay in calling 9-1-1 or the local emergency number, start-

ing CPR and using an AED makes it less likely the victim will survive. Remember, the lay responder is the first link in the victim's cardiac chain of survival.

# Cardiopulmonary Resuscitation (CPR)

It is generally thought that chest compressions create pressure in the chest that causes blood to circulate through the

To find your hand position, find the notch where the lower ribs meet the breastbone *(top)*. Place the heel of your hand on the breastbone, next to your index finger *(middle)*. Place your other hand on top of the first. Use the heel of your bottom hand to apply pressure on the breastbone *(bottom)*.

body. For compressions to be most effective, the victim should be lying on a firm, flat and level surface on his or her back. If a person is in bed, move the person to the floor. CPR does not work as well if the victim is sitting up or is on a soft surface like a mattress.

After determining that a victim does not show signs of circulation, begin chest compressions and rescue breaths. To give chest compressions, kneel beside the victim. Place yourself midway between the head and chest to be able to move easily from giving compressions to giving breaths. Lean over the chest and position your hands. The correct hand and body position lets you give the most effective compressions without tiring you too quickly.

To find the correct hand position, find the notch at the lower end of the victim's breastbone where the ribs meet the breastbone. Slide your middle and index fingers up the edge of the rib cage to the notch where the ribs meet the breastbone. Place your middle finger on this notch. Place your index finger next to your middle finger. Place the heel of one hand above your middle finger. Place your other hand directly on top of it. Try to keep your fingers off the chest by interlocking them together or sticking them out. If you have arthritis or a similar condition in your hands or wrists, you can give compressions by grasping the wrist of the hand positioned on the chest with your other hand.

Compress the chest by pressing down. Then release. You give chest compressions straight down in a smooth, even rhythm. Keeping your elbows locked, arms straight and shoulders directly over your hands and elbows keeps your

**Grasping the wrist of the hand positioned on the chest is an alternate hand position for giving chest compressions.**

arms straight and prevents you from tiring quickly.

When you press down, the weight of your upper body creates the force you need to compress the chest. Push with the weight of your upper body, not with your arm muscles. Push straight down;

**With your hands in place, position yourself so that your shoulders are directly over your hands and your elbows are locked. Press the chest down then release it, keeping a smooth, even rhythm.**

If Person is Not Breathing and Has No Pulse...

# CPR—Adult

Complete "Checking an Unconscious Adult/Child," Pages 32-33.

**Step 1:** **If the victim shows no signs of circulation...** Find hand position on the breastbone.

**Step 2:** Give 15 chest compressions.

**Step 3:** Give 2 rescue breaths.

## Step 4: Do about 3 more cycles of 15 compressions and 2 rescue breaths (for about 1 minute).

## Step 5: Recheck for signs of circulation and breathing for no more than 10 seconds.

## Step 6: If there are no signs of circulation...Continue cycles of 15 compressions and 2 rescue breaths. Recheck for breathing and signs of circulation every few minutes.

**If there are signs of circulation but NO breathing...** GO TO "Rescue Breathing—Adult," Step 1, Pages 50-51.

do not rock your body. Each compression should push the chest down about 2 inches. After each compression, release the pressure on the chest without letting your hands lose contact with the chest. Allow the chest to return to its normal position before you give the next compression.

Keep a steady down-and-up rhythm and do not pause between compressions. Spend half the time going down and half coming up. If your hands slip, find the correct position again. Try not to move them off the chest or change their position. As you do compressions, it helps to count out loud such as: "One, and two, and three…and fifteen" to keep an even pace. You should do compressions at a rate of about 100 compressions per minute.

Give 15 compressions, then reposition the victim's airway. Tilt the head back and lift the chin, then give 2 rescue breaths. Do four continuous cycles of CPR, which should take about 1 minute. Recheck for signs of circulation at the end of the fourth cycle. Check for signs of circulation for no more than 10 seconds. If there are still no signs of circulation, continue CPR. Always recheck for signs of circulation every few minutes. If you find signs of circulation but no breathing, give rescue breaths. If the victim is breathing, place him or her in the recovery position while keeping the victim's airway open. Check for signs of circulation every few minutes until EMS personnel arrive and take over.

## Two-rescuer CPR

If two rescuers at a scene know how to do CPR, one should call 9-1-1 or the local emergency number while the other gives

# When to Stop CPR

**If the victim shows signs of circulation.**

**If another trained person takes over CPR for you.**

**If EMS personnel arrive and take over care of the victim.**

**If you are exhausted and unable to continue.**

**If the scene becomes unsafe.**

CPR. Then one rescuer can help take over when the other one gets tired. When a rescuer gets fatigued, another trained rescuer can either take over compressions **and** rescue breaths or assist by taking over either compressions **or** rescue breaths.

If one rescuer gets tired (often the one giving compressions), he or she may call for a change to take place at the end of the next cycle, such as: "...twelve and, thirteen and, fourteen and change..." for adult CPR. The person giving rescue breaths should simply call for a change when tired. The cycle is then ended with rescue breaths **before** the change takes place. While remaining at **the same side of the victim,** Rescuer 1 (who was giving compressions) moves toward the victim's head to take over rescue breaths but first checks for signs of circulation.

Rescuer 2 (who was giving rescue breaths) moves toward the victim's chest and gets into position to give compressions. If Rescuer 1 does not see or feel signs of circulation, he or she should state "No pulse, continue CPR." CPR is resumed with 15 compressions, then 2 rescue breaths. Signs of circulation should be checked after about the first minute, every few minutes thereafter and when changing positions. Each time signs of circulation are checked, chest compressions must not be stopped for more than 10 seconds during the check. If a second rescuer takes over both chest compressions and rescue breaths for a fatigued rescuer, he or she should check for signs of circulation **for no more than 10 seconds** before beginning CPR.

# Automated External Defibrillation

A person in cardiac arrest needs defibrillation to restore the heart's normal rhythm. A person has the best chance of surviving cardiac arrest if a bystander does CPR and uses an AED within several minutes of the cardiac arrest. EMS personnel can follow up rapidly with further defibrillation, oxygen and intravenous (IV) medication.

An AED is a small machine that analyzes the heart's rhythm and if necessary, tells the responder to deliver a shock to a victim of cardiac arrest. This shock, called defibrillation, may help the heart to reestablish an effective rhythm. If the AED tells the responder "No shock advised," the responder should then check the victim for signs of circulation. If there are no signs of circulation, the responder will need to perform CPR.

AEDs have been placed in many public places such as airports, stadiums and convention centers. Many lives already have been saved because bystanders have used AEDs on victims of cardiac arrest. Contact your local American Red Cross chapter about participating in training on how to use an AED.

# Preventing Coronary Heart Disease

Recognizing a heart attack and getting the necessary care at once may prevent a victim from going into cardiac arrest. However, preventing a heart attack in

# The Brain Speaks

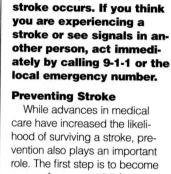

Our brains speak to our bodies through a complex system of nerves, cells and chemicals. In a healthy, well-functioning body, this communication process allows us to swim, enjoy music or tell a joke. However, when the brain does not get enough oxygen to its cells, some may die and cause brain damage, paralysis or even death.

**A disruption of blood flow to a part of the brain that is serious enough to damage brain tissue is called a stroke or a cerebrovascular accident (CVA). Someone suffers a stroke every 53 seconds in the United States, and about 600,000 Americans suffer strokes each year.[16] Most are over the age of 65. Stroke is the third leading cause of death in the United States after heart disease and cancer.[17] Stroke costs the U.S. between $40 to $50 billion per year.[18]**

Stroke is usually caused by a blood clot that forms or lodges in the arteries that supply blood to the brain. Another common cause is bleeding from a damaged artery in the brain. A head injury, high blood pressure, a weak area in an artery wall or fat deposits lining an artery may cause a stroke. A tumor or swelling from a head injury may compress an artery and cause a stroke.

**The signals of a stroke[19] include—**
- **Sudden numbness or weakness of an arm, leg or part of the face, especially on one side of the body.**
- **Sudden confusion, difficulty speaking or inability to understand simple commands or directions.**
- **Sudden trouble seeing in one or both eyes.**
- **Sudden trouble walking, dizziness, loss of balance or coordination.**
- **Sudden severe headache.**

A transient ischemic attack (TIA) is sometimes called a "mini-stroke." Like a stroke, a TIA is caused by reduced blood flow to part of the brain. Unlike a stroke, the signals of a TIA disappear shortly, but the person is not out of danger. Someone who has a TIA has a greater chance of having a stroke in the future.[20] Since you cannot tell a stroke from a TIA, you should call 9-1-1 or the local emergency number for any stroke-like signals.

If you suspect that someone has had a stroke or a TIA, have someone else call 9-1-1 or the local emergency number immediately. If there is fluid or vomit in the victim's mouth, position him or her on one side to allow any fluids to drain out of the mouth. You may have to remove some of the material from the mouth.

If the person is conscious, offer comfort and reassurance. Often he or she does not understand what has happened. Have the person rest in a comfortable position. Do not give the person anything to eat or drink. If the victim is drooling or having trouble swallowing, place him or her on one side to help drain any fluid from the mouth.

**Today medical treatments are available that can reduce or even prevent the long-term effects of having a stroke.[21] However, to be most effective, these treatments must be given as soon as possible after a stroke occurs. If you think you are experiencing a stroke or see signals in another person, act immediately by calling 9-1-1 or the local emergency number.**

## Preventing Stroke

While advances in medical care have increased the likelihood of surviving a stroke, prevention also plays an important role. The first step is to become aware of your own risk factors. Although you cannot control some risk factors like age, family health history, race, ethnicity and sex, you can reduce your overall risk if you are willing to change your behavior to live a healthier lifestyle.

## Controllable Risk Factors
- **High blood pressure—the most important risk factor for stroke**
- **Smoking, especially when combined with use of oral contraceptives**
- **Excessive alcohol intake**
- **History of intravenous drug abuse, especially with cocaine**
- **Diabetes**
- **Heart disease caused by physical inactivity, obesity or high blood cholesterol and lipids**

- Atherosclerosis (hardening of the arteries), especially the carotid arteries in the neck
- High red blood cell level making your blood "thicker"
- Prior stroke or history of TIA's that produce stroke-like symptoms but no permanent damage

You can control many risk factors for stroke. Most important, if you have high blood pressure, talk with your doctor about ways to keep it down. High blood pressure increases your risk of stroke about seven times. High blood pressure puts pressure on arteries and makes them more likely to burst. Even mild high blood pressure can increase your risk of stroke.

Cigarette smoking is another major risk factor for stroke. It increases blood pressure and makes blood more likely to clot. If you do not smoke, do not start. If you do, get help to stop.

A diet high in saturated fats and cholesterol increases your chance of stroke by increasing the possibility of fatty materials building up on the walls of your blood vessels. Eat these foods in moderation.

Regular exercise reduces your chances of stroke by increasing blood circulation, which develops more channels for blood flow. These additional channels provide alternate routes for blood if the primary channels become blocked.

Talk to your health-care provider about your risk of stroke. Ask for support and guidance in making lifestyle changes. Your health-care provider also will be able to offer specific suggestions based on your personal health history on how to reduce your risk of stroke.

the first place is even more effective. There is no substitute for prevention. Heart attacks are usually the result of disease of the heart and blood vessels. Coronary heart disease is the leading cause of death for adults in the United States. It accounts for nearly 500,000 deaths each year.[22]

Coronary heart disease develops slowly. Deposits of cholesterol, a fatty substance made by the body and present in certain foods, build up on the inner walls of the arteries. The arteries gradually narrow. As the arteries that carry blood to the heart get narrower, less oxygen-rich blood flows to the heart. This reduced oxygen supply to the heart can eventually cause a heart attack.

Although a heart attack may seem to strike suddenly, many people live lives that are gradually putting their hearts in danger from coronary heart disease. Because coronary heart disease develops slowly, victims may not be aware of it for many years. Fortunately, it is possible to slow the progress of coronary heart disease by making life-style changes.

Behavior that can harm the heart and blood vessels may begin in early childhood. We may develop a taste for "junk food," which is high in cholesterol and saturated fats but has little real

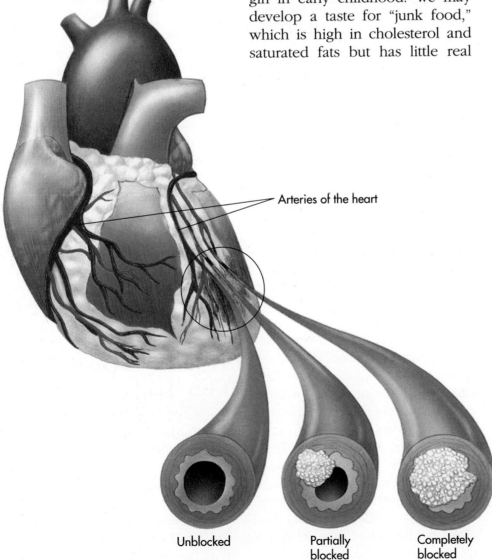

Arteries of the heart

Unblocked

Partially blocked

Completely blocked

**The arteries of the heart supply the heart muscle with blood. A buildup of materials on the inner walls of these arteries reduces the flow of oxygen-rich blood to the heart muscle, causing part of the heart to die. This is called a heart attack.**

nutritional value. Coronary heart disease can begin in the teens especially if those are the years when people begin to smoke. Cigarette smoking greatly contributes to coronary heart disease and to other diseases.

Many things increase a person's chances of developing coronary heart disease. These are called risk factors. Some of them you cannot change. For instance, although more women than men die each year from coronary heart disease in the United States, heart disease generally affects men at younger ages than it does women.

Besides gender, ethnicity also plays an important role in determining the risk for coronary heart disease. African Americans and Native Americans in the United States experience higher percentages of coronary heart disease than do other populations. A history of coronary heart disease in your family also increases your risk.

Many risk factors can be controlled, however. Cigarette smoking, having uncontrolled high blood cholesterol or high blood pressure, being overweight and not exercising regularly all put you at greater risk of heart disease. When you combine one risk factor, like smoking, with others, such as high blood pressure and not enough exercise, your risk of heart attack is much greater.

People are becoming more aware of their risk factors for heart disease and are taking steps to control them. If you also take such steps, you will improve your chances for living a long and healthy life. Remember, it is never too late. Changes you make at any time in your life to lessen your risk will make a difference.

It is important to know how to do CPR and use an AED. The truth remains, however, that the best way to deal with cardiac arrest is to try to prevent it. If you go into cardiac arrest, your chances of surviving are poor. Begin to reduce your risk of coronary heart disease today.

## If Air Does Not Go In

When providing care in a breathing or cardiac emergency, you may not see the victim's chest clearly rise as you give rescue breaths. You might not have tilted the head back far enough. Reposition the victim's airway by tilting the head further back (to ensure that the airway is open) and repeat the breaths. If your breaths

If an unconscious choking victim is pregnant, you can still give chest compressions.

still do not go in, the airway is probably blocked. The airway can become blocked by the tongue falling back in the throat, by food, by an object such as a coin or by fluids such as blood or saliva.

If you have tried to give your initial 2 rescue breaths, repositioned the airway and tried to give 2 rescue breaths again with no success, attempt to clear the airway. This is done by giving chest compressions and then looking for a foreign object. If it is visible, remove the object with your finger and then attempt rescue breaths again.

The most important thing to do is to try to remove the object or move it enough so that you can get air past it into the lungs. First, try to create an artificial cough to force air—and the object—out of

**SKILL SHEET**

**If Air Does Not Go In…**

**IF AN UNCONSCIOUS PERSON'S AIRWAY IS BLOCKED,** it is more important to get air in than to get the object out.

*Complete "Checking an Unconscious Adult/Child," Pages 32-33.*

**Step 1:** **If breaths do not go in...**Tilt the head further back and give 2 rescue breaths again.

**Step 2:** **If breaths still do not go in...Give 15 chest compressions.**

**Step 3:** **Look for a foreign object. If you see one, remove it with your finger.**

## Step 4: Give 2 rescue breaths.

## Step 5: If the breaths still do not go in...Repeat Steps 2-4.

**If the breaths go in...** Check for signs of circulation for no more than 10 seconds.

**If there are no signs of circulation...** GO TO "CPR—Adult," Pages 68-69.

**If there are signs of circulation but NO breathing...** GO TO "Rescue Breathing—Adult," Step 1, Pages 50-51.

**If there are signs of circulation and breathing...** Place the victim in a recovery position.

the airway. To give chest compressions to an unconscious victim whose airway is blocked, you use the same technique as used in CPR. Kneel to the side of the victim and find the correct hand position by finding the notch at the lower end of the victim's breastbone where the ribs meet the breastbone. Slide your middle and index fingers up the edge of the rib cage to the notch where the ribs meet the breastbone. Place your middle finger on this notch. Place your index finger next to your middle finger. Place the heel of one hand above your middle finger. Place your other hand directly on top of it. Try to keep your fingers off the chest by interlocking them together or sticking them out. If you have arthritis or a similar condition in your hands or wrists, you can give compressions by grasping the wrist of the hand positioned on the chest with your other hand.

Position your shoulders over your hands and compress the chest about 2 inches deep. After giving 15 chest compressions, lift the victim's lower jaw and tongue with your fingers and thumb. Look for a foreign object. If you see a foreign object, slide one finger down the inside of the victim's cheek and try to remove it. Be careful not to push the object further down. Give 2 rescue breaths (at this time do not reposition the airway to give rescue breaths). If you still cannot get air into the victim, continue the sequence of 15 chest compressions, foreign object look/removal and 2 rescue breaths. Continue this sequence until the object is removed and the chest clearly rises with rescue breaths, the victim starts breathing on his or her own or EMS personnel arrive and take over.

# Preventing Heart Disease

Coronary heart disease is the leading cause of death for people over the age of 45 living in the United States. Although heart attacks may seem to strike suddenly, most of us make lifestyle choices every day that endanger our hearts. Over time, our choices can result in a heart attack or heart disease.

Scientists have identified factors that increase a person's chances of developing coronary heart disease. These are known as risk factors. Some risk factors for coronary heart disease cannot be changed. For example, men have a higher risk for heart disease at younger ages than women. Having family members who have had coronary heart disease also increases your risk.

Many risk factors for coronary heart disease can be controlled. Smoking, diets high in fats, high blood pressure, obesity, and lack of routine exercise are all linked to increased risk of coronary heart disease. When one risk factor, such as high blood pressure, is combined with other risk factors, the risk of heart attack or stroke is greatly increased. Managing your risk factors for coronary heart disease really works. During the past 20 years, deaths from coronary heart disease have gone down dramatically in the United States, saving as many as 250,000 lives each year!

# Smoking

Cigarette smokers have more than twice the chance of having a heart attack than non-smokers. They have two to four times the chance of cardiac arrest. The earlier a person starts smoking, the greater the risk to his or her health. Giving up smoking rapidly reduces the risk of heart disease. After a number of years, the risk for a person who stopped smoking is the same as the risk for a person who never smoked.

Recent studies indicate that even if you do not smoke, smoking may be increasing your risk of coronary heart disease. Inhaling the smoke of others, called second-hand smoke, may be as dangerous as smoking. You should avoid long-term exposure to high levels of smoke and protect children from this potential danger. If you do not smoke, do not start. If you do smoke, quit.

# Diet

Diets high in saturated fats and cholesterol increase the risk of coronary heart disease. These diets raise the level of cholesterol found in the bloodstream. This increases the chances that cholesterol and other fatty deposits will be deposited on blood vessel walls, reducing blood flow.

Some cholesterol in the body is essential. The amount of cholesterol in the blood is determined by how much your body produces and by the food you eat. Foods high in cholesterol include egg yolks, shrimp, lobster and organ meats such as liver or kidneys.

A more significant contributor to an unhealthy blood-cholesterol level is saturated fat. Saturated fats raise the blood cholesterol level by interfering with the body's ability to remove cholesterol from the blood. Saturated fats are found in beef, lamb, veal, pork, ham, whole milk and whole-milk products.

Rather than eliminating saturated fats and cholesterol from your diet, limit your intake. Moderation is the key. Make changes whenever possible. Substitute low fat or skim milk for whole milk and margarine for butter. Trim visible fat from meat and broil or bake instead of frying. Substitute fish for red meat occasionally. Eat fruits and vegetables for snacks instead of prepackaged or fast food. Read labels carefully. A "cholesterol free" product may actually be high in saturated fat.

# Exercise

Routine exercise has many benefits, including increased muscle tone and weight control. Exercise may also help you survive a heart attack because the increased circulation of blood through the heart develops additional channels for blood flow. If the primary channels that supply the heart are blocked in a heart attack, these additional channels can supply the heart with oxygen-rich blood.

Most of us wish we had more time to exercise. We know that exercise is good for almost every system in our body. But if you have limited time, it is best to build up cardiovascular fitness. Cardiovascular fitness can help you cope with stress, control your weight, ward off infections, improve self-esteem, sleep better and accomplish your personal fitness goals.

To achieve cardiovascular fitness, you must exercise your heart. To do this, you should exercise at least three times a week for 20 to 30 minutes, maintaining your target heart rate for at least 15 minutes. Your target heart rate range is 65 to 80 percent of your maximum heart rate. To find your target heart rate range, subtract your age from 220, then multiply that number by 0.65.

Consider a 40-year-old who wants to exercise at 65 percent of his or her maximum heart rate. The target heart rate would be $(220-40) \times 0.65 = 117$ beats per minute. This person should get his or her pulse rate to 117 beats per minute for at least 15 minutes during the workout.

As you exercise, take your pulse periodically at the wrist or neck. Exercise must be continuous and vigorous to maintain the target heart rate. As you build cardiovascular fitness, you will eventually be able to exercise for longer periods of time and at a higher target heart rate. The "no pain, no gain" theory is not a good approach to exercise. In fact, feeling pain usually means that you are exercising improperly. Be sure to warm up before vigorous exercise and cool down afterwards.

Turn your daily activities into exercise. Walk briskly or bicycle instead of driving. Climb the stairs instead of taking the elevator or escalator. Pedal an exercise bike or use a stair climber while watching TV, listening to music or reading.

If you have not been exercising regularly or have health problems, see your doctor before starting an exercise program.

# Blood Pressure

Uncontrolled blood pressure can damage blood vessels in the heart and other organs. You can often control high blood pressure by losing excess weight and changing your diet. When these are not enough, a doctor can prescribe medications. You should take medications only as prescribed, and only your doctor should adjust them.

High blood pressure has no specific, easily recognized symptoms. It is important to have regular checkups to guard against high blood pressure and its effects. Free blood pressure checks may be available in your community at agencies, hospitals, health fairs or pharmacies.

# Weight

Many adults and children are overweight, some to the point of obesity. Obesity is defined as weighing 20 percent more than your desirable body weight. Obesity contributes to diseases such as heart disease, high blood pressure, diabetes and gall bladder disease. However, body weight is not the main problem. The presence of too much body fat contributes to these diseases. See your doctor for help if you want a measure of your body fat.

Losing weight, especially fat, is no easy task. Weight loss and gain depend on a balance of intake of calories and output of energy. If you take in more calories than you use, you gain weight. If you use more calories than you take in, you lose weight.

Day-to-day weight changes reflect changes in the level of fluids in your body. So if you are watching your weight, pick one day and time each week for your weigh-in. Track your weight loss based on this weekly amount, not on day-to-day differences.

Weight loss should always be combined with daily exercise. Any activity, such as walking to the bus, climbing the stairs, and cleaning the house, uses calories. The more active you are, the more calories you use.

Your eating habits should change as you grow older. If a person eats the same number of calories at the ages of 20 and 40 and maintains the same level of activity, he or she will be considerably heavier at 40 than at 20. It is important as you grow older to eat foods that provide your body with essential nutrients but are not high in calories.

# When Seconds Count:
# children
## & Life-Threatening Emergencies

Unintentional injury is still the number one killer of America's children, with 1 out of 4 children (14 million) injured seriously enough each year to require medical attention.[23] If you are around children frequently, it is likely that you will have to care for a child or infant with an injury or illness. It is important to remember that children are not just small adults.

You might think that, because they are physically smaller, children do not need to breathe as fast as adults or that their hearts do not beat as fast.

# Injury...

## is the leading cause of death of children in the U.S.

Children actually breathe faster than adults and their hearts beat faster. The demands on their little bodies are great. In a breathing or cardiac emergency, children require care that is different from adults. Infants from birth to 1 year of age receive slightly different care from that of children ages 1 to about 8.

In a life-threatening emergency, you must act at once. It may only be a matter of seconds before a child or infant dies. An emergency is life threatening if the child or infant is unconscious, not breathing, having trouble breathing, shows no signs of circulation or is bleeding severely.

Before widespread immunization programs began about 40 years ago, infectious diseases, such as polio and diphtheria, were the main killers of children. Now injury is the leading cause of death in children in the United States. The numbers are staggering. In 1998, 9,854,000 visits were made to U.S. hospital emergency departments because of injuries to children.[24] The six most common types of childhood injuries are motor vehicle-related injuries, drownings, fires and burns, suffocations, falls and firearms.[25]

Most injuries can be prevented. If they were, childhood deaths and disabilities would be greatly reduced. As children grow and develop and as they are exposed to different environments, they become vulnerable to different injuries and illnesses. Adults have the responsibility of making the environment safe for children. This can be done by—
- Keeping children away from things that might harm them.
- Staying near children so that you can act quickly in an emergency.
- Following safety rules yourself and teaching them to children.

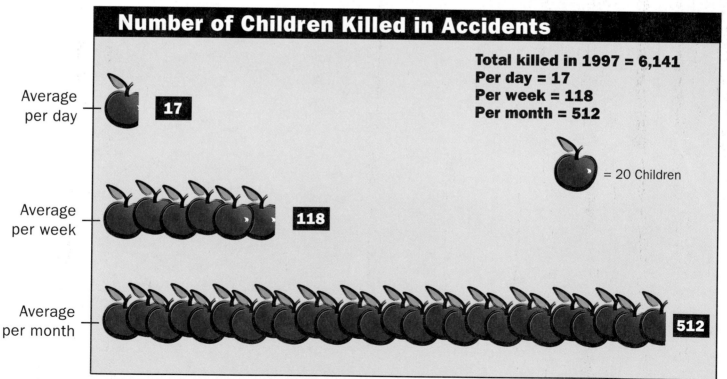

**Number of Children Killed in Accidents**

Total killed in 1997 = 6,141
Per day = 17
Per week = 118
Per month = 512

= 20 Children

Average per day — 17

Average per week — 118

Average per month — 512

Source: National Center for Health Statistics, 1997 Edition.

# Why Always Get Hurt

Children are naturally curious about people and objects in the world around them. They spend much of their time exploring and learning. At the same time, their small bodies are growing quickly and becoming more mobile. A child's developing body, however, is less skilled and more prone to injury than an adult's. A child's body proportions are also different from an adult's. For example, a child's head is quite large and heavy compared with the rest of the body. This puts children at greater risk for head injuries. Children's eyesight and hearing take time to fully develop. Thus they are often injured by traffic that they do not hear or see while walking or cycling.

One way infants learn about their world is by putting objects in their mouths. They also grasp and pull with their hands and wiggle and move their bodies. All of these actions can lead them into danger. The infant who can pick up a button or coin can put it in his or her mouth and choke. The infant who can pull a cup from a coffee table can be burned by hot liquid. The infant who can roll over can roll off a bed and suffer a head injury. Infants face many new dangers as they learn to roll, crawl, stand, climb and walk.

Infants cannot recognize dangers and it is up to adults to protect them. Often, protecting them is as simple as removing the dangers. A bottle of furniture polish stored under a kitchen sink could poison a curious crawler. The danger can easily be removed by storing the polish in a locked cabinet where the child cannot reach it.

Like infants, toddlers and older children are always exploring and trying new things. Because they can walk, they tend to get into more trouble than infants do. They learn to copy adult behaviors and begin to understand how things work. They use words to ask for things and talk to other people, yet they lack judgment and understanding of potential risks. For instance, children cannot judge the depth of water.

Children are often injured when they are left alone, even for a few minutes. Young children need constant adult guidance and supervision, but the amount and kind of supervision needed changes as children grow and develop.

You can teach children safety in two ways. First, you can set an example of safe behavior by acting safely yourself. Second, you can encourage children to act safely by giving them simple, clear instructions about what they should and should not do. For example, teach children to always buckle their safety belts. Explain to them how a safety belt protects them from getting hurt. Teach them that they should not touch a hot stove and explain the meaning of the word hot. Remember to be patient. It takes time to learn safe behaviors and make them a habit.

For more information on keeping children safe, contact:

**U.S. Consumer Product Safety Commission**
**Washington, DC 20207-0001**
**http://www.cpsc.gov**
**(800) 638-CPSC**
**(800) 638-8270 (TTY/TTD)**
Evaluates the safety of products sold to the public. Provides printed materials on consumer product safety topics on request.

**National Maternal and Child Health Clearinghouse**
**http://www.nmchc.org**
**(888) 434-4MCH**
Provides information and printed materials on maternal and child health.

# GENERAL SAFETY RULES

Here are some basic safety rules you can follow to protect children:

**Properly install car seats and use them for all motor vehicle travel involving infants and smaller children.**

**Buckle up larger children in the back seat of motor vehicles.**

**Always watch children in or near water.**

**Never keep loaded guns in your home.**

**Use gates on stairs.**

**Keep plastic bags, cords and small objects away from young children.**

**Call the Poison Control Center if you think a child has been poisoned.**

**Have a plan for dealing with emergencies.**

**Check your home for fire and burn dangers.**

## Breathing Emergencies

The human body needs a constant supply of oxygen to stay alive. During breathing, air enters the nose and mouth. The air travels down the throat, through the windpipe and into the lungs. This pathway from the nose and mouth to the lungs is called the airway. As you might well imagine, a child's airway is much smaller than an adult's. But as for an adult, the airway must be open for air to go into the lungs. In the lungs the oxygen in the air is picked up by the blood. The heart pumps the blood through the body. The blood flows through the blood vessels, taking the oxygen to the brain and to all other parts of the body.

A breathing emergency happens when air cannot travel freely and easily into the lungs. Some emergencies are life threatening because they greatly cut down on the oxygen the body receives or cut off the oxygen entirely. The heart will soon stop beating and blood will no longer move through the body. Unless the brain gets oxygen within minutes, brain damage or death will occur.

A breathing problem so severe that it threatens the victim's life is a breathing emergency. It is very important to recognize breathing emergencies in children and infants and to act before the heart stops beating. This is often the key to saving a child's or infant's life.

Adult hearts frequently stop beating because they are diseased. For example, heart attacks are a common result of coronary heart disease. Children's hearts, however, are usually healthy. When a child's heart stops, it is usually the result of a breathing emergency. If the child cannot breathe properly, not enough oxygen gets into the blood. This starves the heart of oxygen and the heart soon stops beating. Children whose hearts stop beating rarely survive. Of the few who do, most suffer permanent brain damage.

Most cardiac emergencies in children can be prevented. There are three main ways to do this. One way is to keep children from being injured. A second is to make sure children have proper medical care. A third is to learn to recognize the early signals of a breathing emergency and know what to do about such an emergency.

Breathing emergencies can be caused by injury or illness. Injury or disease in areas of the brain that control breathing can disturb or stop breathing. A major cause of breathing emergencies is choking on a piece of food or a small object.

Damage to the muscles or bones of the chest can make breathing painful or difficult. Electric shock and drowning can cause breathing to stop. Allergic reactions may make the airway swell shut. Reactions to poisons, anxiety, excitement and conditions such as asthma can all cause breathing emergencies.

Asthma is a condition that narrows the air passages and makes breathing difficult. Asthma may be triggered by a reaction to food, pollen, medications, insect stings, chemical irritants or pollutants. A typical signal of asthma is wheezing when the child breathes out. A child's chest may look larger than normal because air becomes trapped in the lungs. Normally asthma is controlled with medica-

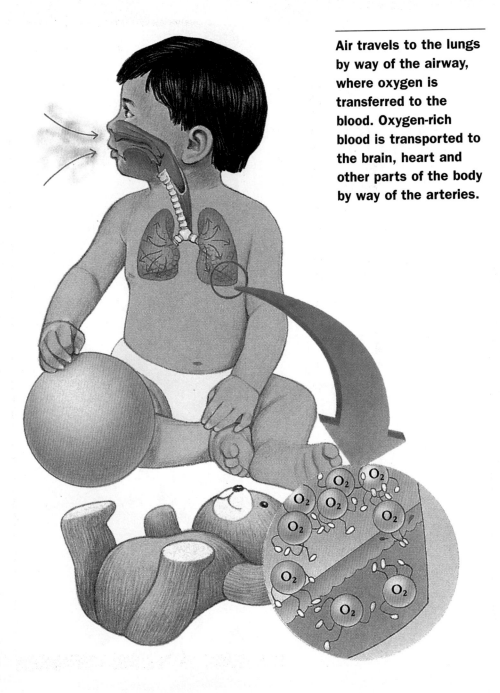

## Adults are responsible...
### for making sure children are safe.

Air travels to the lungs by way of the airway, where oxygen is transferred to the blood. Oxygen-rich blood is transported to the brain, heart and other parts of the body by way of the arteries.

Unless the brain gets oxygen... brain damage or death will occur within minutes.

tions that open the airway and make breathing easier.

Hyperventilation occurs when a child breathes faster than normal. Causes include fear or anxiety, injuries, illnesses such as high fever and diabetic emergencies. It can also result from asthma or exercise. A typical signal of hyperventilation is shallow, rapid breathing. Despite trying hard to breathe, children who are hyperventilating say that they cannot get enough air or that they are suffocating. Therefore they are often frightened and confused. They may say that they feel dizzy or that their fingers and toes feel numb or tingly.

A severe allergic reaction can cause the airway to swell and restrict breathing. It may result from insect stings, food or medications, such as penicillin. If you know a child is allergic to certain substances, keep the child away from them. A physician may recommend that the child or an adult

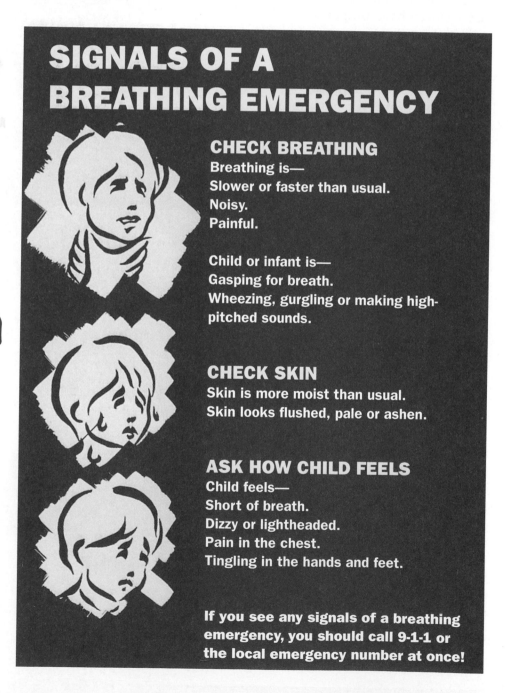

# SIGNALS OF A BREATHING EMERGENCY

## CHECK BREATHING
Breathing is—
Slower or faster than usual.
Noisy.
Painful.

Child or infant is—
Gasping for breath.
Wheezing, gurgling or making high-pitched sounds.

## CHECK SKIN
Skin is more moist than usual.
Skin looks flushed, pale or ashen.

## ASK HOW CHILD FEELS
Child feels—
Short of breath.
Dizzy or lightheaded.
Pain in the chest.
Tingling in the hands and feet.

If you see any signals of a breathing emergency, you should call 9-1-1 or the local emergency number at once!

guardian carry medication to reverse the reaction. Sometimes this medication comes packaged in a "pen" so that the medication can be injected into the body. Ask the parent or guardian if the child needs help with the medication and help to administer it if requested.[26]

Signals of allergic reaction may develop very quickly. They include a rash, a feeling of tightness in the chest and throat and swelling of the face, neck and tongue. The child may feel dizzy or confused. If not cared for at once, severe allergic reactions can become life threatening.

Even though there are many causes of breathing emergencies, you do not have to know the exact cause to respond. You do need to be able to recognize the signals of a breathing emergency and take action fast!

## Recognizing Breathing Emergencies

You are most likely to have to care for a conscious child or infant who is having trouble breathing. You will probably be able to identify a breathing problem by watching and listening to the way the child or infant breathes. A child who can talk may be able to tell you what is wrong.

Normal breathing is easy and quiet. Children should not have to work at breathing. Breaths should be regular and breathing should not be painful.

There are many signals of possible breathing emergencies. They might not be the same for all children. Children and infants may look as if they cannot catch their breath or they may gasp for

# When a child's heart stops... it is usually the result of a breathing emergency...

air. They may be breathing faster or slower than normal. Their breaths may be deeper or more shallow than usual. They may make unusual noises, such as wheezing or gurgling, or high-pitched sounds.

The child's skin may also signal that something is wrong. At first, the child's skin may be more moist than usual and look flushed. Later it may look pale or ashen as the oxygen level in the blood falls.

A child having a breathing problem may feel dizzy or light-headed. The child may complain that his or her chest hurts and that

his or her hands and feet are tingling. The child may be frightened. Any of these signals could indicate a breathing emergency. If you are unsure or cannot tell if it is a life-threatening emergency, call 9-1-1 or the local emergency number.

A child who can talk may be able to tell you that he or she finds it difficult to breathe. For infants and very young children, though, you must use your own judgment based on how the child looks and the way he or she is breathing. If you see any signals of a breathing emergency, you should get emergency medical care at once.

# Make Your Home Safe for Kids

## Storage Areas

YES/NO  Are pesticides, detergents and other household chemicals kept out of child's reach?

YES/NO  Are tools kept out of child's reach?

## General Safety Precautions Inside the Home

YES/NO  Are stairways kept clear and uncluttered?

YES/NO  Are stairs and hallways well lit?

YES/NO  Are safety gates installed at tops and bottoms of stairways?

YES/NO  Are guards installed around fireplaces, radiators or hot pipes and wood-burning stoves?

YES/NO  Are sharp edges of furniture cushioned with corner guards or other material?

YES/NO  Are curtain cords and shade pulls kept out of child's reach?

YES/NO  Are fire extinguishers installed where they are most likely to be needed?

YES/NO  Are smoke alarms installed and in working order? Are batteries changed at least every 6 months?

YES/NO  Do you have an emergency plan to use in case of fire? Does your family practice this plan?

YES/NO  Is the water set at a safe temperature? (A setting of 120°F or less prevents scalding from tap water in sinks and in tubs. Let the water run for 3 minutes before testing it.)

YES/NO  If you have a gun, is it locked in a place where your child cannot get it? Are bullets stored and locked separately from guns?

YES/NO  Are all purses, handbags, brief cases and so on, including those of visitors, kept out of child's reach?

YES/NO  Are all poisonous plants kept out of child's reach?

YES/NO  Is a list of emergency phone numbers posted near telephones?

YES/NO  Is a list of instructions posted near telephones for use by children or babysitters?

## Bathroom

YES/NO  Are the toilet seat and lid kept down when the toilet is not in use?

YES/NO  Are cabinets equipped with safety latches and kept closed?

YES/NO  Are all medicines in child-resistant containers and stored in a locked medicine cabinet?

YES/NO  Are shampoos and cosmetics stored out of child's reach?

YES/NO  Are razors, razor blades and other sharp objects kept out of child's reach?

YES/NO  Are hair dryers and other appliances stored away from sink, tub or toilet?

YES/NO  Does the bottom of tub or shower have non-slip surfacing?

YES/NO  Is the child always watched by an adult while in the bathroom?

## Kitchen

- **YES/NO** Do you cook on back stove burners when possible and turn pot handles toward the back of the stove?
- **YES/NO** Are hot dishes kept away from the edges of tables and counters?
- **YES/NO** Are hot liquids and foods kept out of child's reach?
- **YES/NO** Are knives and other sharp items kept out of child's reach?
- **YES/NO** Is the highchair placed away from stove and other hot appliances?
- **YES/NO** Are matches and lighters kept out of child's reach?
- **YES/NO** Are all appliance cords kept out of child's reach?
- **YES/NO** Are cabinets equipped with safety latches?
- **YES/NO** Are cleaning products kept out of child's reach?
- **YES/NO** Do you test the temperature of heated food before feeding the child?

Use this checklist to spot dangers in your home. When you read each question, circle either the "Yes" box or the "No" box. Each "No" shows a possible danger for you and your family. Work with your family to remove dangers and make your home safer.

## Child's Room

- **YES/NO** Is child's bed or crib placed away from radiators and other hot surfaces?
- **YES/NO** Are crib slats no more than 2 3/8 inches apart?
- **YES/NO** Does the mattress fit the sides of the crib snugly?
- **YES/NO** Is paint or finish on furniture and toys nontoxic?
- **YES/NO** Is the child's clothing, especially sleepwear, flame resistant?
- **YES/NO** Does the toybox have secure lid and safe-closing hinges?
- **YES/NO** Are electric cords kept out of child's reach?
- **YES/NO** Are the toys in good repair?
- **YES/NO** Are toys appropriate for the child's age?

## Outside the Home/Play Areas

- **YES/NO** Is trash kept in tightly covered containers?
- **YES/NO** Are walkways, stairs and railings in good repair?
- **YES/NO** Are walkways and stairs free of toys, tools and other objects?
- **YES/NO** Are sandboxes and wading pools covered when not in use?
- **YES/NO** Are nearby swimming pools enclosed with a fence that your child cannot easily climb over? Is the backyard pool separated from the home's entrance by a fence?
- **YES/NO** Is playground equipment safe? Is it assembled according to the manufacturer's instructions?

## Parents' Bedroom

- **YES/NO** Are space heaters kept away from curtains and flammable materials?
- **YES/NO** Are cosmetics, perfumes and breakable items stored out of child's reach?
- **YES/NO** Are small objects, such as jewelry, buttons and safety pins, kept out of child's reach?

## CHILD SAFETY IQ

HEALTH CHECK

- ☐ Do you buckle your child into an approved automobile safety seat in the back seat even when making short trips?
- ☐ Do you teach your child safety by behaving safely in your own everyday activities?
- ☐ Do you supervise your child whenever he or she is around water and maintain fences and gates that act as barriers to water?
- ☐ Have you checked your home for potential fire hazards? Are smoke detectors installed and working? Have you installed a carbon monoxide alarm?
- ☐ Are all poisonous substances, such as cleaning supplies, medicines and plants, kept out of a child's reach?
- ☐ Are foods and small items that can choke a child kept out of reach?
- ☐ Have you inspected your home, day-care center, school, babysitter's home or wherever your child spends time for potential safety and health hazards?
- ☐ Do you keep guns and ammunition stored separately and locked up?

# CARING FOR

# BREA

# EMERG

# CHILDREN WITH

# THING

# ENCIES

Recognizing the signals of breathing emergencies and caring for them are often keys to preventing other emergencies. Any breathing trouble may signal the beginning of a life-threatening condition.

## IF A CHILD OR INFANT HAS TROUBLE BREATHING

If a conscious child or infant is having trouble breathing, help him or her rest in a comfortable position. Sitting usually makes breathing easier. Make sure someone has called 9-1-1 or the local emergency number for help. Stay with the child or infant until EMS personnel arrive.

Remember that children who are having trouble breathing may have trouble talking. Talk to any bystanders who may know the child's problem. Children often answer yes-or-no questions by nodding or shaking their heads. Keep checking breathing and skin appearance. Try to reduce any anxiety that might have contributed to the breathing problem by comforting him or her. Help keep the child or infant from getting chilled or overheated. Help give any medication prescribed for a particular condition.

**If a conscious infant or child is having trouble breathing, support him or her in a sitting position.**

**Care for an infant is slightly different than care for a child.**

**Infant
(0-1 YEAR)**

**Child
(1-8 YEARS)**

If the child or infant is breathing rapidly (hyperventilating) and you are sure it is caused by emotion, such as excitement, not injury or illness, try to get the child to relax and breathe slowly. Reassurance is often enough to correct hyperventilation. If the child's breathing still does not return to normal or if the child becomes unconscious from hyperventilating, call or have someone call 9-1-1 or the local emergency number right away.

If you recognize the signals of a breathing emergency and can provide care, you may be able to prevent the condition from developing into a more serious emergency. If the child stops breathing, he or she may die without immediate care.

The care for infants and children with breathing emergencies is similar. But as you read earlier, some of the techniques are a little different because infants and children vary in size. In general, skills that are described for a child should be used for a child from about age 1 to about age 8. Infant skills should be used for those under 1 year of age. A general guideline is to perform infant skills on a child or infant about the length of your thigh or whom you can comfortably support with your forearm and hand. Perform child skills on a child who is larger than this.

## IF A CONSCIOUS CHILD IS CHOKING

Choking is a common childhood injury that can lead to death. When a child is choking, the airway is partly or completely blocked, usually by food or other small objects. Children often choke while they are eating and

# CARING FOR BREATHING DIFFICULTY

Call the local emergency phone number for help.

Help the child or infant rest in the position easiest for breathing.

Comfort the child or infant.

Keep checking breathing.

Make sure the child or infant does not get chilled or overheated.

Give any prescribed medication.

# PREVENTING CHOKING

**Don't leave small objects, such as buttons, coins, and beads, within an infant's reach.**

**Have children sit in a high chair or at a table while they eat.**

**Do not let children eat too fast.**

**Give infants soft food that they do not need to chew.**

**Make sure that toys are too large to be swallowed.**

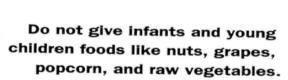

**Do not give infants and young children foods like nuts, grapes, popcorn, and raw vegetables.**

**Make sure that toys have no small parts that could be pulled off.**

**Cut foods a child can choke on easily, such as hot dogs, into small pieces.**

**Supervise children while they eat.**

can choke on a very small piece of food. Also, children cannot or do not always chew food well. Some foods that an adult can eat easily can cause a child to choke.

Tasting is one way children explore their world. Young children, especially those under the age of three, often put objects, such as coins, beads and toys, in their mouths. This is normal, but it can lead to choking.

A choking child can quickly stop breathing, lose consciousness and die. Therefore, it is very important to recognize when a child needs first aid for choking. One of the signals of choking is coughing. Sometimes a child who is choking will cough forcefully. At other times the child may cough weakly or make a high-pitched sound while coughing. A child who is not able to breathe

**Clutching the throat with one or both hands is universally recognized as a distress signal for choking.**

Encourage a choking child who is coughing forcefully to continue coughing.

If a child is choking and cannot cough, speak or breathe, give quick, upward thrusts to the abdomen, just above the belly button, until the object is forced out.

**If Child is Unable to Speak, Cough, or Breathe....**

or cough at all may panic and clutch his or her throat with one or both hands.

If the child is coughing forcefully, the airway is partially blocked but the child is still able to get some air. Stay with the child. Tell the child to keep on coughing. The coughing may clear the airway. If the child does not stop coughing soon or does not cough up the object, call 9-1-1 or the local emergency number for help.

If the child is coughing weakly or is making a high-pitched sound or if the child cannot speak, breathe or cough, the airway is completely blocked. You must give first aid right away. Try to remove the object that is blocking the airway by creating an artificial cough. With one of your legs between the child's feet for support, wrap your arms around the child's waist. Make a fist with one hand and place it against the middle of the child's abdomen, just above the belly button. Grab your fist with your other hand. Give quick upward thrusts into the abdomen until the object is forced out. If you are too tall to give abdominal thrusts while standing, kneel behind the child.

Stop giving thrusts as soon the child coughs up the object or

starts to breathe or cough. Watch the child and make sure that he or she is breathing freely again. Even after the child coughs up the object, the child may have breathing problems that will need medical attention. Also, abdominal thrusts may cause injuries. For these reasons, you should call 9-1-1 or the local emergency number so that the child can be checked by an appropriate health-care provider. Do this even if the child seems to be breathing well.

**Step 1:** **Check the scene and the victim…**
Ask the victim if he or she is choking. Identify yourself and ask the parent or guardian if you can help. If the victim is coughing forcefully, encourage continued coughing.

**Step 2:** **If the victim cannot cough, speak or breathe…**
Have someone else call 9-1-1 or the local emergency number.

**Step 3:** **Give abdominal thrusts…**
Stand behind the victim. Place the thumb side of your fist against the middle of the victim's abdomen. Grasp your fist with your other hand and give quick, upward thrusts.

**If the victim becomes unconscious, call 9-1-1, or the local emergency number, if it has not been done… GO TO "Unconscious Choking— Child," Step 3, Pages 110-111.**

## IF A CHILD IS NOT BREATHING

A child may stop breathing because of illness, injury or a blocked airway. A child who is not breathing is getting no oxygen. The body can function only for a few minutes without oxygen before body systems begin to fail.

Rescue breathing is a way of breathing air into a person to supply the oxygen he or she needs to survive. A child who is unconscious and not breathing but shows signs of circulation needs rescue breathing.

Begin by tilting the head back and lifting the chin to move the tongue away from the back of the throat. This opens the airway. Place your ear next to the child's mouth. Look, listen and feel for breathing for about 5 seconds. If you cannot see, hear or feel any

signs of breathing, pinch the child's nose shut, take a breath and make a tight seal around the child's mouth with your mouth. Breathe slowly and gently into the child until you see the chest clearly rise. Do this twice. Each breath should last about 1½ seconds. Pause between each breath to let the air flow back out. Watch the child's chest clearly rise each time you breathe into the child to be sure that your breaths are actually going in.

If, at any time during your care, you do not see the child's chest clearly rise as you give rescue breaths, you might not have tilted the head far enough back. Reposition the victim's airway by tilting the head further back (to ensure that the airway is open) and repeat the breaths. If your

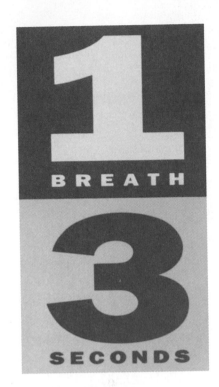

**If there are signs of circulation (e.g., a pulse) but the child is not breathing, give 1 breath about every 3 seconds.**

If a child stops breathing, you must breathe for him or her. This is called rescue breathing.

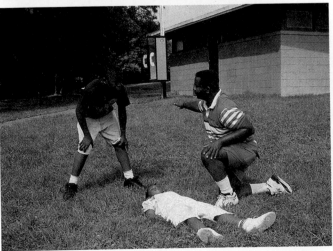

If someone is with you when you discover an unconscious child, have that person phone for help while you continue to give care.

**1 MINUTE**

**CALL FAST: If you are alone and the child is not breathing and does not have a history of heart problems, give care for about 1 minute before calling 9-1-1 or the local emergency number.**

If the child is small enough, carry him or her to the phone while you continue to give breaths.

breaths still do not go in, the airway is probably blocked. The airway can become blocked by the tongue falling back in the throat, by food, by an object such as a coin or by fluids such as blood or saliva. You will learn how to clear a blocked airway in a later lesson ("If Air Does Not Go In").

Check for signs of circulation. Signs of circulation include normal breathing, coughing or movement in response to rescue breaths and a pulse. Check for a child's pulse by finding the Adam's apple and sliding your fingers toward you and down into the groove at the side of the

child's neck. Check for signs of circulation **for no more than 10 seconds.** If there are signs of circulation but the child is still not breathing, give 1 breath about every 3 seconds. A good way to time the breaths is to count out loud, such as: "one one-thousand," take a breath on "two one-thousand" and breathe into the child on "three one-thousand" to keep an even pace.

After about 1 minute of rescue breathing (about 20 breaths), recheck for signs of circulation and breathing. Recheck for signs of circulation **for no more than 10 seconds.** If the child still shows signs of circulation but is not breathing, continue rescue breathing. Check for signs of circulation every minute when giving rescue breathing.

Continue rescue breathing until one of the following happens:

- The scene becomes unsafe.
- The child begins to breathe on his or her own.
- You are too exhausted to continue.
- Another trained responder takes over for you.

Call 9-1-1 or the local emergency number for help if a child is unconscious. If someone is with you when you discover an unconscious child, have that person phone for help immediately. This way, you can continue checking the child and give rescue breathing or any other necessary care at once. If you are alone and you find a child unconscious and not breathing, give rescue breathing for about 1 minute before calling 9-1-1 or your local emergency number. This delay in phoning allows you to give breaths that will get oxygen into the child and prevent the heart from stopping. If the child is small

**If vomiting occurs, turn the child on his or her side and wipe the mouth clean.**

enough, carry him or her to the telephone while continuing to give rescue breaths.

When you are giving rescue breathing, you want to avoid getting air in the child's stomach instead of the lungs. This may happen if you breathe into the child too long, too hard or do not open the airway far enough.

To avoid getting air in the child's stomach, keep the child's head tilted back. Breathe *slowly and gently* into the child, just enough to make the chest clearly rise. Each breath should last about 1½ seconds. Pause between breaths long enough for the air in the child's lungs to come out and for you to take another breath.

Air in the stomach can make the child vomit and cause serious complications. When an unconscious child vomits, the contents of the stomach can get into the lungs and block breathing. Air in the stomach also makes it harder for the diaphragm, the large muscle that controls breathing, to move. This makes it harder for the lungs to fill with air.

Even when you are giving rescue breathing properly, the child may vomit. If this happens, roll the child onto one side and wipe the mouth clean. If possible, use latex gloves, gauze or even a handkerchief when you clean out the mouth. Then roll the child on his or her back again and continue with rescue breathing.

Sometimes you might not be able to make a tight enough seal over a child's mouth. For example, the child's jaw or mouth may be injured or shut too tightly to open. If you cannot make a tight seal over the mouth, you can breathe into the nose. With the head tilted backward, close the child's mouth by gently pushing on the chin.

Seal your mouth around the child's nose and breathe into the nose. If possible, open the child's mouth between breaths to let the air out.

Finally, you should suspect head, neck or back injuries if a child has fallen from a height or has been in a motor vehicle accident. Do not remove a child from a car seat. If a child is wearing a helmet, do not remove it. If you suspect such an injury, try not to move the child's head, neck and back.

If you need to open the airway, do so using the *jaw-thrust maneuver.* For the jaw-thrust maneuver, place one hand on each side of the child's head, resting your elbows on the surface on which the victim is lying. Grasp the angles of the child's lower jaw and lift with both hands. If the lips close, you can pull back on the lower lip with your thumb. Close the child's nostrils during rescue breathing by

**For mouth-to-nose breathing, close the child's mouth, seal your mouth around the child's nose and breathe into the nose.**

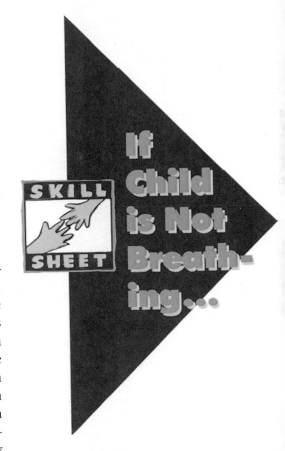

**If you suspect head, neck or back injury, try to open the airway by using the jaw-thrust maneuver.**

# Rescue Breathing—Child

*Complete "Checking an Unconscious Adult/Child," Pages 32-33.*

**Step 1:** **If the child shows signs of circulation but is NOT breathing...**Keep the airway open. Seal your mouth tightly around the child's mouth and pinch the nose shut. Give 1 rescue breath about every 3 seconds. **Do this for about 1 minute (20 breaths).**

**Step 2:** **Recheck for signs of circulation and breathing about every minute.**

**If there are no signs of circulation...
GO TO "CPR—Child," Step 1,
Pages 106-107.**

For a child, check for a pulse at the side of the neck.

placing your cheek tightly against them. This will usually allow air to pass into the lungs. Remember that if a child is not breathing, his or her greatest need is for air.

## IF A CHILD DOES NOT SHOW SIGNS OF CIRCULATION

Your check of an unconscious child includes checking for breathing and signs of circulation. If the child is not breathing, it is possible that his or her heart will stop beating. Checking for signs of circulation can tell you whether or not the child's heart has stopped. Check for signs of circulation **for no more than 10 seconds**. For a child, check for a pulse at the side of the neck. If the child does not show signs of circulation, you should start CPR.

CPR has two parts. One part is chest compressions. When you give chest compressions, press down and let up on the lower half of the breastbone. The second part of CPR is rescue breaths. When you give CPR, you alternate chest compressions and rescue breaths.

When you breathe into the mouth of a child who has stopped breathing, you are keeping the lungs supplied with oxygen. The oxygen in the lungs goes into the blood. When you compress the chest, you keep blood flowing throughout the child's body. The blood carries oxygen to the brain, heart and other parts of the body. CPR keeps blood flowing through the body, especially to the brain.

You must start CPR as soon as possible after the child's heart stops beating. If brain cells do not get oxygen, they begin to die after about 4 minutes. Starting CPR right away increases the chances that the child will survive.

Once you have decided that a child needs CPR, you must put yourself and the child in the correct position. Place the child on his or her back, on a firm, flat and level surface. Kneel beside the child's chest. Keep the child's head tilted back with one hand placed on the child's forehead. Using your hand nearest the child's feet, trace up the child's rib cage to the notch with two fingers and place the heel of your hand on the child's breastbone in the middle of the chest above the

To give compressions, keep the head tilted back with one hand and place the heel of your other hand on the lower half of the breastbone. Press the chest down and then release it in a smooth, even rhythm.

**If a child is not breathing and does not show signs of circulation, give cycles of 5 compressions and 1 breath.**

notch. Push down and let up five times. Each compression should be about 1½ inches deep. These 5 compressions should take about 3 seconds. Count out loud, such as: "one, and two, and three,…" to help you maintain an even and regular rhythm.

After giving 5 compressions, you must get oxygen into the child's lungs. With the child's head tilted back, lift the chin and give 1 rescue breath (for about 1½ seconds) until the chest clearly rises. Repeat cycles of 5 compressions and 1 rescue breath for about 11 more cycles (1 minute). Then recheck for signs of circulation for no more than 10 seconds. In a child, check for a pulse by finding the Adam's apple and sliding your fingers toward you and down into the groove at the side of the child's neck. If the child shows no signs of circulation, continue CPR until help arrives. Recheck every few minutes for breathing and signs of circulation when giving CPR.

## TWO-RESCUER CPR

If two rescuers at the scene know how to do CPR, one rescuer should call 9-1-1 or the local emergency number while the other gives CPR. Then one rescuer can take over when the other one gets tired. When a rescuer gets tired, another trained rescuer can either take over both compressions **and** rescue breaths or take over either compressions **or** rescue breaths.

If one rescuer gets tired (often the one giving compressions), he or she may call for a change to take place at the end of the next cycle, such as: "...two, and three, and four, and five and change…" for child CPR. The person giving the rescue breaths should simply call for a change when tired. The cycle is then ended with the rescue

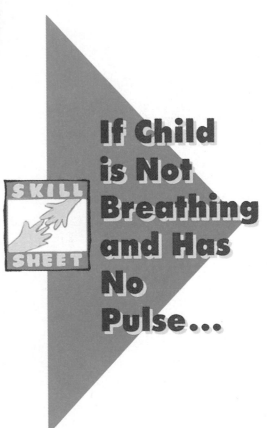

If Child is Not Breathing and Has No Pulse...

# CPR—Child

*Complete "Checking an Unconscious Adult/Child," Pages 32-33.*

**Step 1:** **If the child shows no signs of circulation...**

Find hand position on the breastbone.

**Step 2:** Give 5 chest compressions.

**Step 3:** Give 1 rescue breath...

**Step 4:** Do about 11 more cycles of 5 compressions and 1 rescue breath (for about 1 minute).

**Step 5:** Recheck for signs of circulation and breathing for no more than 10 seconds.

**Step 6:** If there are no signs of circulation...

Continue cycles of 5 compressions and 1 rescue breath. Recheck for breathing and signs of circulation every few minutes.

**If there are signs of circulation but NO breathing...
GO TO "Rescue Breathing—Child," Step 1, Pages 102-103.**

breath **before** the change takes place. While remaining at **the same side of the child,** Rescuer 1 (who was giving compressions) moves toward the child's head to take over rescue breaths but first checks for signs of circulation.

Rescuer 2 (who was giving rescue breaths) moves toward the child's chest and gets into position to give compressions. If Rescuer 1 does not see or feel signs of circulation, he or she should state "No pulse, continue CPR." CPR is resumed with 5 compressions, then 1 rescue breath. Signs of circulation should be checked after about the first minute, every few minutes thereafter and when changing positions. Each time signs of circulation are checked, chest compressions must not be stopped for more than 10 seconds during the check. If a second rescuer takes over both chest compressions and rescue breaths, he or she should check for signs of circulation **for no more than 10 seconds** before beginning.

## IF AIR DOES NOT GO IN

When providing care for breathing and cardiac emergencies, you may find that an unconscious child's chest does not clearly rise as you give rescue breaths. If you did not tilt the head back far enough, the child's tongue may be blocking the throat. Reposition the child's airway and give 2 more rescue breaths. If you still cannot breathe air into the child, the child's airway is probably blocked. The airway can be blocked by food, a small object, such as a toy or coin, or fluids, such as blood and saliva. Tell someone to call 9-1-1 or the local emergency number while you provide care.

The most important thing to do is to try to remove the object or move it enough so that you can get air past it into the lungs. Use the same technique for chest compressions that you used in CPR. First, try to create an artificial cough to force air—and the object—out of the airway. To do this, place one hand on the child's forehead to maintain an open airway and with your hand closest to the child's feet, find the correct hand position for chest compressions. Find the notch at the lower edge of the child's rib cage. Slide your middle and index fingers up the edge of the rib cage to the notch where the ribs meet the breastbone. Place your middle finger on this notch. Place your index finger next to your middle finger. Place the heel of this hand on the breastbone next to where your index finger was. Position your shoulder straight over your compression hand with your elbow "locked." Give 5 chest compressions about 1½ inches deep at a rate of about 100 compressions per minute.

Look to see if a foreign object is in the child's mouth. If you can see the object, slide a finger down the inside of the child's cheek and try to remove the object.

Then give 1 rescue breath. If the child's chest does not clearly rise, continue cycles of 5 chest compressions, foreign object look/removal and 1 rescue breath until the scene becomes unsafe, the child starts breathing on his or her own, you are too exhausted to continue or EMS personnel arrive and take over.

If you do clear the airway and can breathe into the child, give a second rescue breath and then check for breathing and signs of circulation **for no more than 10**

If at any time you find that your rescue breaths will not go in, use the same technique that you used for CPR. Give 5 chest compressions.

Look for an object in the throat. Slide a finger down inside of the cheek and try to remove the object only if you can see it.

Open the airway and attempt to give 1 breath. If the breath goes in, immediately give one more breath and check for signs of circulation.

SKILL SHEET

If Air Does Not Go In...

**seconds.** If the child is not breathing but shows signs of circulation, continue rescue breathing. If there is no breathing and no signs of circulation, begin CPR.

If your first attempts to clear the airway do not succeed, do not give up. The longer the child goes without oxygen, the more the muscles of the throat will relax.

This will make it more likely you will be able to remove the object or breathe past it.

If the child starts breathing on his or her own, keep the airway open, place the child in the recovery position and continue to check breathing until EMS personnel arrive and take over.

# Unconscious Choking—Child

*Complete "Checking an Unconscious Adult/Child," Pages 32-33.*

**Step 1:** **If breaths do not go in...** Tilt the head further back and give 2 rescue breaths again.

**Step 2:** **If breaths still do not go in...Give 5 chest compressions.**

**Step 3:** **Look for a foreign object. If you see one, remove it with your finger.**

**Step 4:** **Give 1 rescue breath.**

**Step 5:** **If the breath still does not go in...**

Repeat Steps 2-4.

**If the breath goes in, give another breath then...**Check for signs of circulation for no more than 10 seconds.

**If there are no signs of circulation... GO TO "CPR—Child," Pages 106-107.**

**If there are signs of circulation but NO breathing...GO TO "Rescue Breathing—Child," Step 1, Pages 102-103.**

**If there are signs of circulation and breathing...Place the child in a recovery position.**

# Caring for Infants
## With Breathing Emergencies

*C*are for infants (birth to 1 year) and children with breathing and cardiac emergencies is similar. You should check to see if an unconscious infant:

- Has an open airway.
- Is breathing.
- Shows signs of circulation.
- Is bleeding severely.

An easy way to recall what you need to check, is to remember ABC: Airway (open the airway), Breathing (check for breathing) and Circulation (check for signs of circulation and severe bleeding).

Care differs in a few areas because infants and children vary in size. In general, the skills presented here should be used for an

infant under 1 year of age. If you are uncertain of the infant's age, use your own judgment. If an infant is too long or too heavy for you to support him or her on your arm and hand, especially if the infant is choking, use the technique for a child.

## If a Conscious Infant Is Choking

Choking is a major cause of death and injury in infants. One reason is that infants learn about their world by putting objects in their mouths. Small objects, such as pebbles, coins, beads and parts of toys, are dangerous if an infant puts them in the mouth. Infants also often choke because it takes a long time to develop their eating skills. Infants can easily choke

on some foods that an adult can eat, such as nuts, grapes, popcorn or sliced hotdogs.

To prevent choking, never let an infant eat alone. Never prop up a bottle for an infant to drink alone. Always stay with an infant during meals or snacks. Cut food into small pieces. Do not give an infant foods, such as nuts, that could lodge in the airway. If you suspect that an infant has an object in his or her mouth, check with your fingers and remove it. Regularly check floors, rugs and other places for pins, coins and other small objects that an infant might pick up and put in his or her mouth.

Like a child who is choking, a choking infant can quickly stop breathing, lose consciousness and die. If the infant is coughing forcefully, allow the infant to continue to cough. Watch the infant carefully. If the infant cannot cough, cry or breathe, have someone call 9-1-1 or the local emergency number for help. To clear the blocked airway of a conscious infant, you will need to give back blows and chest thrusts.

To do this, position the infant on your arm, with your hand supporting the infant's head. With your other hand, strike the infant between the shoulder blades 5 times. Turn the infant over face-up on your forearm, supporting the head, neck and back. Locate the correct hand position for chest thrusts by imagining a line running across the chest between the infant's nipples. Place the ring finger (or index finger) of your hand on the infant's breastbone just below this imaginary line. Place the pads of the two fingers next to your ring finger (or index finger) on the infant's breastbone. Lift your ring finger (or index finger). Give 5

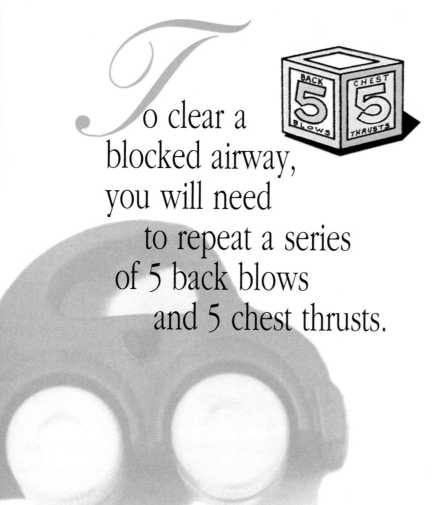

To clear a blocked airway, you will need to repeat a series of 5 back blows and 5 chest thrusts.

chest thrusts, about one per second. Each thrust should be about ½–1 inch deep. Turn the infant facedown again and repeat back blows followed by chest thrusts. Keep the infant's head lower than the chest.

Stop as soon as the object is coughed up or the infant starts to breathe or cough. Watch the infant and make sure that he or she is breathing freely again. Call 9-1-1 or the local emergency number if you have not already done so. The

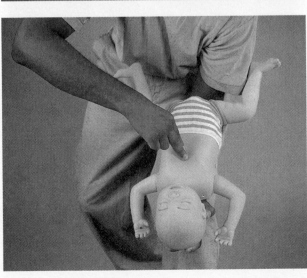

**Position the infant face-down on your forearm so that the head is lower than the chest.**
**Give 5 back blows between the shoulder blades** *(top).*
**Turn the infant onto his or her back** *(middle).*
**Give 5 chest thrusts in the center of the breastbone** *(bottom).*

SKILL SHEET

If Infant is Unable to Cry, Cough, or Breathe...

# Conscious Choking—Infant

**Step 1:** Check the scene and the infant...
Identify yourself and ask the parent or guardian if you can help.

**Step 2:** If the infant cannot cough, cry or breathe...Have someone else call 9-1-1 or the local emergency number.

**Step 3:** Give 5 back blows with the heel of your hand between the shoulder blades.

**Step 4:** Position the infant face-up on your forearm.

**Step 5:** Place two fingers on the center of the breastbone just below the nipples and give 5 chest thrusts...

Repeat Steps 3-5 until the foreign object is coughed up or the infant becomes unconscious.

**If the infant becomes unconscious... GO TO "Unconscious Choking—Infant," Step 3, Pages 126-127.**

*An* infant who is not breathing needs rescue breathing. Give 1 breath about every 3 seconds.

infant should be taken to the hospital emergency department to be checked by a health-care provider. Do this even if the infant seems to be breathing well.

## If an Infant Is Not Breathing

When an infant stops breathing, his or her body can function for only a few minutes without oxygen before body systems begin to fail. Like a child, an infant who is not breathing but shows signs of circulation needs rescue breathing immediately. Rescue breathing provides the oxygen the infant needs to survive. You discover whether you need to give rescue breaths when you check the infant's breathing. Open the infant's airway by tilting the head back with one hand and lifting the chin with the other hand. Look, listen and feel for breathing for about 5 seconds. You do not need to tilt an infant's head back very far to open the airway.

If the infant is not breathing, you will have to give rescue breaths. Because an infant's mouth is so small, you should take a breath and then, using a breathing barrier, cover the infant's mouth and nose instead of just covering the mouth as you would for a child. Give 2 rescue breaths. Breathe slowly and gently into the infant only until you see the chest clearly rise. Each breath should last about 1½ seconds. Pause in between rescue breaths to let the air flow back out. Watch the chest clearly rise each time you breathe in to be sure that your rescue breaths are actually going in.

If, at any time during your care, you do not see the infant's chest clearly rise as you give rescue breaths, you might not have tilted the head back far enough.

**To give rescue breaths to an infant, seal your mouth over the infant's mouth and nose.**

# Rescue Breathing—Infant

*Complete "Checking an Unconscious Infant," Pages 34-35.*

**Step 1:** If the infant shows signs of circulation but is NOT breathing...Keep the airway open, seal your lips tightly around the infant's mouth and nose. Give 1 rescue breath about every 3 seconds for about 1 minute (20 breaths).

**Step 2:** Recheck for signs of circulation and breathing about every minute...

Continue rescue breathing as long as the infant shows signs of circulation but is **NOT** breathing.

**If there are no signs of circulation...**

**GO TO "CPR — Infant," Step 1, Pages 122-123.**

Reposition the victim's airway by tilting the head a little further back (to ensure that the airway is open) and repeat the breaths. If your breaths still do not go in, the airway is probably blocked. The airway can become blocked by the tongue falling back in the throat, by food, by an object such as a coin or by fluids such as blood or saliva. You will learn how to clear a blocked airway in a later lesson ("If Air Does Not Go In").

Check for signs of circulation **for no more than 10 seconds.** Signs of circulation include normal breathing, coughing or movement in response to rescue breaths and a pulse. In an infant, check for a pulse by pressing your first two fingers against the bone on the inside of the infant's upper arm between the elbow and the shoulder. If the infant is not breathing but shows signs of circulation, continue rescue breathing. Give 1 rescue breath about every 3 seconds. A good way to time the breaths is to count out loud, such as: "one one-thousand," take a breath yourself on "two one-thousand," and breathe into the infant on "three one-thousand" to keep an even pace. Remember to breathe slowly and gently. Breathing too hard or too fast can force air into the infant's stomach.

After 1 minute of rescue breathing (about 20 breaths), recheck the infant for breathing and signs of circulation. Check for signs of circulation **for no more than 10 seconds.** If the infant still shows signs of circulation but is not breathing, continue rescue breathing until—

- The scene becomes unsafe.
- The child begins to breathe on his or her own.
- You are too exhausted to continue.
- Another trained responder takes over for you.

Check for breathing and signs of circulation every minute when giving rescue breathing.

## If An Infant Does Not Show Signs of Circulation

An infant who is not breathing and does not show signs of circulation needs CPR. Signs of circulation include normal breathing, coughing or movement in response to rescue breaths and a pulse. Feel for an infant's pulse on the inside of the upper arm, between the infant's elbow and shoulder. Start CPR if you cannot find signs of circulation after checking for no more than 10 seconds.

To give CPR, place the infant on his or her back on a firm, flat and level surface, such as the floor or a table. If you must move the infant to the telephone when you call for help, the hard surface can be your hand or forearm, with your palm supporting the infant's back. Locate the correct hand position for chest compressions by imagining a line running across the chest between the infant's nipples. Place the index finger of your hand closest to the infant's feet on the infant's breastbone just below this imaginary

**Feel for an infant's pulse on the inside of the arm, between the infant's elbow and shoulder.**

line. Place the pads of the two fingers next to your index finger on the infant's breastbone. Lift your index finger. If you feel the notch at the end of the infant's breastbone, move your fingers slightly toward the infant's head.

Use the two fingers to compress the infant's chest down 5 times about ½ to 1 inch deep and at a rate of at least 100 compressions per minute. These 5 compressions should take less than 3 seconds. Count out loud, such as: "one, two, three, four, five,…" to help to keep a regular and even rhythm.

After giving 5 compressions, give 1 rescue breath (about 1½ seconds). Then begin compressions again. Repeat cycles of 5 compressions and 1 rescue breath for about 19 more cycles (1 minute). Then recheck for signs of circulation for no more than 10 seconds. If there are still no signs of circulation, continue with cycles of 5 compressions and 1 rescue breath until help arrives. Check every few minutes for breathing and signs of circulation.

Ask someone to call 9-1-1 or the local emergency number as soon as you find out that the infant is unconscious. If you are

**An infant who is not breathing and does not show any signs of circulation needs CPR. Alternate giving 5 chest compressions and 1 breath.**

**If Infant is Not Breathing and Has No Pulse…**

alone with an infant who is known to be at risk for heart problems, call 9-1-1 first and then begin CPR; otherwise provide 1 minute of care then call. If possible, carry the infant to the telephone so that you can begin CPR immediately while talking with the dispatcher or after hanging up.

**The hard surface of your hand and forearm can be used to support an infant during CPR if you have to move to a phone.**

# CPR—Infant

*Complete "Checking an Unconscious Infant," Pages 34-35.*

## Step 1: If the infant shows no signs of circulation...

Place one hand on the infant's forehead to keep the airway open. Find finger position in the center of the breastbone by placing two fingers just below the nipples.

## Step 2: Give 5 chest compressions.

## Step 3: Give 1 rescue breath...

**Step 4:** Do about 19 more cycles of 5 compressions and 1 rescue breath for about 1 minute.

**Step 5:** Recheck for signs of circulation and breathing for no more than 10 seconds.

**Step 6:** If there are NO signs of circulation...Continue cycles of 5 compressions and 1 rescue breath. Recheck for breathing and signs of circulation every few minutes.

If there are signs of circulation but NO breathing...GO TO "Rescue Breathing—Infant," Step 1, Pages 118-119.

# SIDS

"**F**or the first few months, I would lie awake in bed at night and wonder if she was still breathing. I mean you just never know. I couldn't get to sleep until I checked on her at least once." This is how one mother described her first experience with parenting.

Sudden Infant Death Syndrome (SIDS) is the sudden, unexpected and unexplained death of apparently healthy babies. It is the major cause of death of infants between the ages of 1 month and 1 year. In the United States, SIDS, previously called crib death, is responsible for the death of about 3,000 infants each year.[27]

Because it cannot be predicted or prevented, SIDS causes many new parents to feel anxious. With no warning signals, a sleeping infant can stop breathing and never wake again. Parents and other family members of SIDS victims often have trouble dealing with this traumatic event. Researchers are working to find the cause(s) of SIDS. At this time, several risk factors—characteristics that occur more often in SIDS victims than in normal babies—have been discovered. Yet these risk factors are not causes and cannot be used to predict which infants will die. For example, 90 percent of SIDS deaths occur in infants under 6 months of age, so being in this age group is a risk factor. Boys are at higher risk than girls. Other risk factors for SIDS include exposing an infant to smoking during and after pregnancy, first pregnancy under 20 years of age, several children already born to the mother, a baby with a low birth weight or born premature and a baby with a low growth rate during the mother's pregnancy. Twins and higher multiples are also at increased risk.[28]

## Some basic facts about SIDS:

- Ninety percent of SIDS deaths occur while the infant is asleep.
- SIDS deaths can occur between the ages of 2 weeks and 18 months. Ninety five percent of deaths occur between 2 and 4 months of age.
- The majority of SIDS deaths occur in fall and winter.
- Between 30 and 50 percent of SIDS victims have minor respiratory or gastrointestinal infections at the time of death.
- SIDS occurs slightly more often in boys than in girls.

For more information, call the National SIDS Resource Center at (703) 821-8955, ext. 249.

It is important for pregnant women to practice healthy behaviors while pregnant. They should get proper prenatal care, eat a balanced diet, not smoke or drink alcoholic drinks and get adequate rest and exercise.

Important steps can also be taken to reduce the likelihood of SIDS after an infant's birth. Infants who sleep on their stomachs during the night or naptime have an increased risk of SIDS.[29] Make sure that *everyone* who comes into contact with your infant—you, grandparents and other relatives, child-care providers, babysitters—know always to place an infant on his or her back at night or naptime, using a firm mattress in a safety-approved crib or bassinet. This recommendation has helped to reduce the SIDS rate by 42 percent in the last decade. That means saving 2,000 infant lives a year.[30] Do not wait to talk about the importance of placing an infant on his or her back to sleep. Your infant's life could depend on it.

## If Air Does Not Go In

When giving care for breathing and cardiac emergencies, if the infant's chest does not clearly rise, the infant's airway is probably blocked. The infant's tongue or an object may block it. If the infant was left alone with a bottle to drink, fluids may be blocking the airway. Tell someone to call 9-1-1 or the local emergency number for help while you provide care.

You must clear the blockage immediately. First, reposition the infant's airway by tilting the head further back and lifting the chin. Try to give 2 rescue breaths again. If the rescue breaths still do not go in, you must assume there is something blocking the airway.

Use the same technique for chest compressions that you used in CPR. If you have not already done so, place the child on a firm, flat and level surface. Maintain an open airway with one hand on the infant's forehead and find the correct hand position with your other hand. Locate the correct hand position for chest compressions by imagining a line running across the chest between the infant's nipples. Place the index finger of your hand closest to the infant's feet on the infant's breastbone just below this imaginary line. Place the pads of the two fingers next to your index finger on the infant's breastbone. Lift your index finger. If you feel the notch at the end of the infant's breastbone, move your fingers slightly toward the infant's head. Use two fingers to compress the infant's chest down 5 times about ½–1 inch deep and at a rate of at least 100 compressions per minute.

Look in the infant's mouth for a foreign object by grasping the infant's tongue and lower jaw between your thumb and fingers and lifting the jaw upward. If you can see the foreign object, remove it with your little finger. Then give 1 rescue breath to try to get air into the infant's lungs.

If the chest does not clearly rise, continue cycles of 5 chest compressions, foreign object look/removal and 1 rescue breath until the infant coughs the object up and begins to breathe or cough on his or her own or EMS personnel arrive and take over.

If you do clear the airway and can breathe into the infant, give a second rescue breath and then check for breathing and signs of circulation for no more than 10 seconds. If the child is not breathing but shows signs of circulation, continue rescue breathing. If there is no breathing and no signs of circulation, begin CPR.

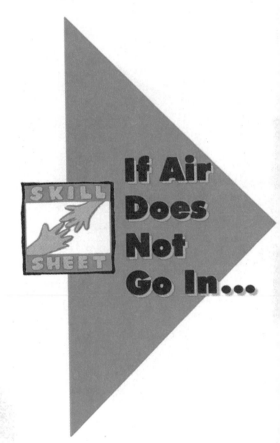

SKILL SHEET

If Air Does Not Go In...

*If you are unable to breathe into an infant, the airway is probably blocked.*

# Unconscious Choking—Infant

*Complete "Checking an Unconscious Infant," Pages 34-35.*

**Step 1:** **If breaths do not go in...**Tilt the infant's head further back and give 2 rescue breaths again.

**Step 2:** **If breaths still do not go in...**

Find finger position on the breastbone and give 5 chest compressions.

**Step 3:** **Look for a foreign object.**

If you see one, remove it with your little finger.

## Step 4: Give 1 rescue breath.

## Step 5: If the breath still does not go in...Repeat Steps 2-4.

**If the breath goes in...**

Give another breath and check for signs of circulation.

**If there are no signs of circulation...GO TO "CPR—Infant," Step 1, Pages 122-123.**

**If there are signs of circulation but NO breathing...GO TO "Rescue Breathing—Infant," Step 1, Pages 118-119.**

**If there are signs of circulation and breathing...**

Continue monitoring ABCs.

The wail of sirens breaks the sleepy afternoon stillness. A police car suddenly pulls to a stop on the shady street and an officer goes into a house. An ambulance drives up and two paramedics dart into the house. Another ambulance quickly arrives and still others head toward the house. For a few moments all is quiet. Suddenly several people emerge from the house carrying a stretcher. On it is a body—not very large. Paramedics cluster around the body, frantically trying to save the child's life. They slide the stretcher into the ambulance. A distraught woman runs after them. She turns to the police officer next to her. "I don't know where he found the gun," she chokes. "My husband keeps it in his desk. It couldn't have been loaded."

# INJURIES

Injury is one of our nation's most important health problems. Most of us will have a significant injury at some time in our lives. In the few minutes it takes you to read this information, 10 people will be killed and almost 400 will suffer disabling injuries. Besides the cost in grief and pain, these injuries will amount to $469 billion in lost income, medical expenses, property damage, insurance and other costs.[31]

## Causes of Injury

Injuries that damage, disable and kill are caused by different types of force. For example, a blow to the chest can break ribs. A bullet that travels through skin and muscle can strike a blood

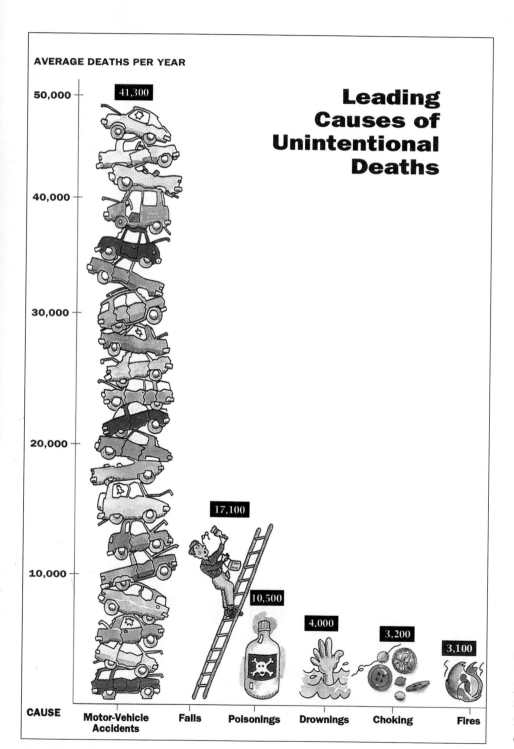

**AVERAGE DEATHS PER YEAR**

# Leading Causes of Unintentional Deaths

| | | | | | | |
|---|---|---|---|---|---|---|
| 41,300 | | | | | | |
| | 17,100 | | | | | |
| | | 10,500 | | | | |
| | | | 4,000 | 3,200 | 3,100 | |

**CAUSE**: Motor-Vehicle Accidents · Falls · Poisonings · Drownings · Choking · Fires

National Safety Council Injury Facts, 2000.

M ost of us will have a significant injury at some time in our lives.

vessel and cause serious bleeding within the body.

Sometimes, a force causes an injury to an area in the body away from where it strikes. This happens, for example, when you fall and try to break the fall with an outstretched hand and the force of the impact travels up your arm, injuring your shoulder.

Moving your body in certain ways also causes injuries. Even movements as simple as stepping off a curb or turning to reach for an out-of-the-way object can cause injury. Suddenly contracting or tightening a muscle, or group of muscles, can also cause injury. These types of muscle injuries commonly happen in sports activities, sometimes as a result of not warming up or cooling down enough.

You can also be injured by the energy from heat, chemicals, radiation and electricity, which all cause burns. Thousands die each year from fires and burns. They are the sixth leading cause of unintentional deaths. Most of these fatal injuries happen at home. Fires cause 83 percent of all deaths from burns.[32] Smoking is the leading cause of fire deaths in the home overall, but in the winter months heating equipment contributes significantly to the number of fire-related deaths.[33] Of an estimated 1.25 million burn injuries per year in the U.S., over 600,000 require medical care in a hospital emergency department.[34]

## Reducing Your Risk of Injury

How does this information relate to you? What are your chances of injury? What can you do to reduce your risk of injury?

People of certain ages are injured more often than others. In-

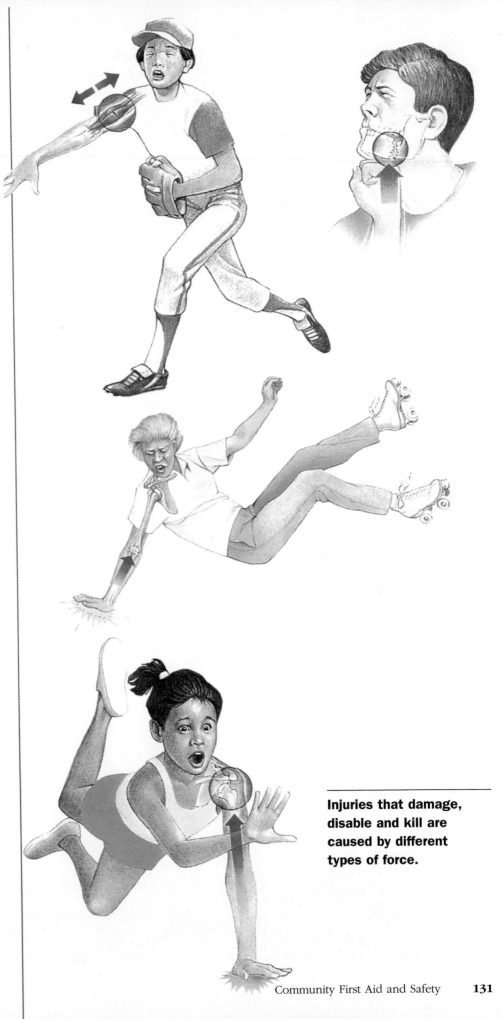

Injuries that damage, disable and kill are caused by different types of force.

### Total Cost of Injury

Cost of accidents by class, 2000

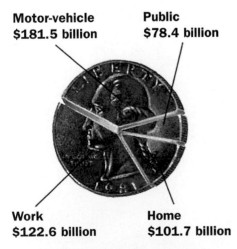

**Motor-vehicle** $181.5 billion

**Public** $78.4 billion

**Work** $122.6 billion

**Home** $101.7 billion

**Total Cost: $469.0 billion***

*Duplication between motor-vehicle and work was $15.2 billion.
National Safety Council, *Injury Facts*, 2000

jury rates are higher for people under 45. Injuries resulting in death occur most often among people aged 15 to 24. Men are more likely to be injured than women.

Many people believe that injuries just happen. They believe that those who are injured are just unfortunate victims of circumstance, but this is not true. Overwhelming evidence exists that injuries, like disease, do not just happen. Rather, many injuries are predictable, preventable events resulting from the way people interact with the potential dangers in the environment.

Your chances of being injured are influenced most by what you do.

There are three general strategies for preventing injury:
- Persuade people at risk to change their behavior.
- Require people at risk to change their behavior.
- Provide automatic protection products designed to reduce the risk of injury.

Although laws that require you to take safety measures, such as wearing safety belts, are moderately effective, the most successful injury-prevention strategy is the protection built into the product. Automatic protection, such as airbags in motor vehicles, does not allow people to make choices.

Typically, behaviors of members of high-risk groups tend to be the hardest to influence. For

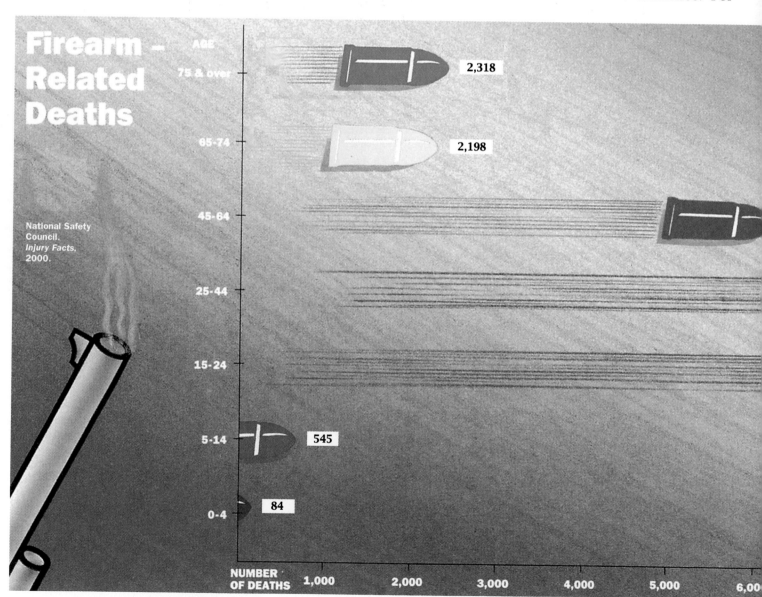

**Firearm – Related Deaths**

National Safety Council, *Injury Facts*, 2000.

AGE

| 75 & over | 2,318 |
| 65-74 | 2,198 |
| 45-64 | |
| 25-44 | |
| 15-24 | |
| 5-14 | 545 |
| 0-4 | 84 |

NUMBER OF DEATHS   1,000   2,000   3,000   4,000   5,000   6,00 example, despite the overwhelming number of traffic deaths in the 15-to-19 age group, teenagers are less likely than adults to wear seat belts.

Many people view laws that require certain behaviors as an infringement of their rights—even though the laws are intended to protect them from injury. Product designs are also difficult to influence because many manufacturers are reluctant to commit the resources for design changes. For instance, the evidence in favor of safety belts was available many years ago. However, it took over 20 years to get a federal regula-

Insurance Institute for Highway Safety

**Automatic protection, such as airbags in motor vehicles, does not allow people to make choices about safety.**

**F**irearm-related deaths continue to be a major public health problem in the United States. Despite an estimate that more than 44 million Americans own more than 192 million firearms,[35] the incidence of firearm-related injury and death has declined over the last five years. It is important to learn about safe and responsible firearm ownership. Many Americans are increasingly concerned about firearms used to injure or cause death intentionally, including the use of firearms in suicides and multiple-victim violence.

**I**n 1997, more than 32,000 people died from firearm-related deaths in the United States; another 64,000 people were injured and treated for gunshot wounds in hospital emergency departments.[36] Over 85 percent of these deaths were males. Among this population, those men between the ages of 20-24 are most at risk for firearm-related death, with males 15-19 years of age and 25-29 years of age forming the second level of at-risk populations.[37] As infrequent but highly publicized acts of violence at schools, jobs and religious sites occur, responses are needed because the violence **happens, not** because it captures public attention.

National Safety Council Injury Facts, 2000.

**12,688**

**8,112**

7,000    8,000    9,000    10,000    11,000    12,000    13,000    14,000    15,000

# WATCH YOUR BAC!

**W**hat's *your* BAC? Not a question you would usually be able to answer, but if you are suspected of driving drunk, the police will find the answer by taking a blood, breath or urine sample and analyzing it. BAC stands for blood alcohol concentration. The test result is expressed as a blood alcohol concentration percentage.

In the United States, each state has set a legal limit for BAC. States punish those who choose to drive drunk with fines, loss of license or jail. In most states, a driver with a BAC of 0.10 percent or more is considered to be driving while intoxicated (DWI).[38] For a 140-pound person, reaching this blood alcohol level takes about three drinks in 1 hour.

One drink equals 12 oz. of beer, 5 oz. of wine or 1½ oz. of hard liquor.

Although BAC limits have been established for lawful driving, a lower BAC can still impair the physical and mental abilities you need to drive safely. Your judgment, coordination and reaction times are all dulled by alcohol.

Researchers estimate that the risk of being involved in a fatal crash may be at least eight times higher for a drunk driver than a sober one.

Motor vehicle accidents are a major cause of death from injury in the United States. In 1998, 30 percent of all traffic fatalities involved intoxicated drivers or pedestrians, according to the National Highway Traffic Safety Administration. Of the 12,456 people killed, 70 percent were intoxicated; the other 30 percent were victims of other people's intoxication.[39] Traffic deaths and crashes involving alcohol occur most often to people who are 18 to 24 years of age. Young people are often less used to alcohol and take more risks.

### NUMBER OF DRINKS

| BODY WEIGHT | 1 | 2 | 3 | 4 | 5 |
|---|---|---|---|---|---|
| 100 | .04 | .09 | .15 | .20 | .25 |
| 120 | .03 | .08 | .12 | .16 | .21 |
| 140 | .02 | .06 | .10 | .14 | .18 |
| 160 | .02 | .05 | .09 | .12 | .15 |
| 180 | .02 | .05 | .08 | .10 | .13 |
| 200 | .01 | .04 | .07 | .09 | .12 |

The amount of alcohol in mixed drinks varies considerably, depending on the recipe and type of liquor used.

Figures are rounded to nearest .01. BACs shown are approximate, since they can be affected by factors other than weight.

**0 to .04**
Not legally under the influence. Impairment possible.

**.05 to .09**
State laws vary. Mental and physical impairment noticeable.

**.10 and above**
Presumed intoxicated in all 50 states.

National Clearinghouse for Alcohol Information

**Think before you drink.**

● Exercise your right to say "no thanks" to the first drink or to any other drink.

● Be honest with yourself—realize that even one drink can increase your risk of injuring yourself or someone else.

● Switch to nonalcoholic beverages like juice or soda when you have reached your limit.

● Never drink and drive—choose a driver who agrees not to drink. Take public transportation or stay overnight.

For more information about how to prevent alcohol-related deaths and injuries, contact your local chapters of Mothers Against Drunk Driving (MADD) by accessing the national office of MADD at www.madd.org/ Contact Students Against Destructive Decisions (SADD) by calling the national office at 1-800-787-5777.

## Reducing Your Risk of Injury

**T**ake measures that can decrease the risk of injury for you and others.

**T**hink safety—be alert and avoid potentially harmful conditions or activities that increase your injury risk.

**T**ake precautions such as wearing protective helmets, padding and eyewear for appropriate recreational activities.

**A**lways buckle your seatbelt when driving or riding in motor vehicles.

**L**et your state and congressional representatives know that you support legislation that ensures a safer environment for us all.

tion requiring automobile manufacturers to install automatic restraints by 1990.

Although there are some injury factors that you can do little about, there are others that you directly control. For example, drinking alcohol is a primary cause of many injuries and deaths, especially from motor vehicle accidents. Many people who die from falls, drowning, fires and firearm-related accidents have more than the legal limit of alco-

hol in their blood. Alcohol is a factor in about 42 percent of motor vehicle accidents, 45 percent of fire fatalities, 38 percent of drowning deaths and 46 percent of homicides.[40,41]

The American Trauma Society contends that, if all the existing information about prevention were applied, the injury rate could be reduced by 50 percent, with most of the gains made for children and young adults, who are most frequently injured.[42]

Injuries do not just happen. For the most part, they are predictable and preventable. If you have not already done so, answer the "Injury Prevention IQ Quiz." The questionnaire will help heighten your awareness of conditions or situations around you that may lead to injury. It may help you reduce your risk of injury, as well as risk to others.

If existing information about prevention were applied, the injury rate could be reduced by 50 percent.

**E**ach year in the United States, thousands of people will die, millions will be injured and over 469 billion dollars[43] will be spent, all needlessly. The cause...many injuries that could have been prevented.

## Mark "yes" or "no" next to the following questions:

**[Y/N]** Do you wear a safety belt when driving or riding in a motor vehicle?

**[Y/N]** Do you refrain from driving after drinking alcoholic beverages?

**[Y/N]** If you own a gun, do you keep it unloaded and locked in a safe place? Are thc bullets stored separately?

**[Y/N]** Do the stairs where you live have handrails?

**[Y/N]** Do you use a stepladder or sturdy stool to reach high, out-of-reach objects?

**[Y/N]** Do you have adequate lighting in halls and stairways?

**[Y/N]** Do you use good lifting techniques when lifting objects?

**[Y/N]** Do you wear a helmet when using a bicycle, motorcycle, scooter, roller blades or skateboard?

**[Y/N]** Do you wear a lifejacket when participating in activities on or near the water?

**[Y/N]** Do you wear safety protection (e.g., goggles and hearing protection) and follow equipment safety recommendations when operating power tools?

HEALTH CHECK

INJURY PREVENTION IQ QUIZ

## If you answered "no" to any of these questions, consider that in the United States—

- Forty-two percent of all deaths from unintentional injuries are a result of motor vehicle accidents.[44]

- Alcohol use is a factor in about 38 percent of all motor vehicle fatalities.[45]

- About 1,000 people die each year of unintentional firearm-related deaths; the deaths often result from improper handling, accessibility to children and lack of safety mechanisms.[46]

- Falls account for the largest number of preventable injuries for persons over 75 years of age.[47]

- Injuries to the back make up 27 percent of all disabling injuries in the workplace.[48]

- About 22 percent of all motor vehicle fatalities are related to bicycle, pedestrian and motorcycle casualties.[49] Increasing helmet usage has reduced the number of fatalities.

- In 1997, there were about 4,000 deaths resulting from drowning. Over 46 percent of drowning victims are between the ages of 15 and 44.[50]

- Death rates for unintentional injuries have dropped for almost all age groups in the last decade in the U.S.; however, the rate has increased by 7 percent for those 75 years of age and older.[51]

# CUTS, SCRAPES & BRUISES

**A**n infant falls and bruises his arm while learning to walk. A toddler scrapes her knee while learning to run. A child needs stitches in his chin after he falls off the monkey bars on the playground. A teenager gets a black eye in a fist fight. A college student suffers a sunburn during a weekend at the beach. An adult cuts his hand while working in a woodshop. What do all these injuries have in common? They are all soft tissue injuries.

## A CONTINUOUS JOURNEY

There are about 60,000 miles of blood vessels in your body. These vessels act as a road map, directing blood to all parts of the body. As long as your heart beats, blood will flow through a continuous circuit of blood vessels known as arteries, veins and capillaries.

These blood vessels vary in diameter. The larger the vessel, the more blood that can flow through it. During rest, the heart pumps about 5 liters of blood per minute through the blood vessels. During exercise, the blood vessels handle as much as six times this amount. This requires the blood vessels to be able to expand.

Arteries are large blood vessels that carry blood from the heart to all parts of the body. Because the blood in the arteries is closer to the pumping action of the heart, blood in the arteries travels faster and under greater pressure than blood in capillaries and veins. Blood flow in the arteries pulses with the heartbeat. Therefore bleeding from the arteries is very fast and heavy. Arterial blood is usually bright red and, because it is under pressure, it spurts from the wound. This is one easily recognizable signal of severe bleeding.

Veins return blood from the body to the heart. Bleeding from the veins is slower, steadier and easier to control than arterial bleeding. Veins are damaged more often because they are closer to the skin's surface. Venous blood is dark red.

Capillaries are tiny blood vessels near the skin. They transfer oxygen and other nutrients to the body's cells. Bleeding from capillaries is usually slow and clots easily. The blood is not as bright a red as blood from the arteries. Bleeding from scrapes and shallow cuts is from capillaries.

---

Soft tissues are the layers of skin and the fat and muscle beneath the skin. Any time the soft tissues are damaged or torn, the body is threatened. Injuries may damage the soft tissues at or near the skin's surface or deep in the body. Severe bleeding can occur at the skin's surface and under it, where it is harder to detect. Germs can get into the body through a scrape, cut or puncture and cause infection.

Burns are a special kind of soft tissue injury. Like other types of soft tissue injury, burns can damage only the top layer of skin or the skin and the layers of fat, muscle and bone beneath.

An injury to the soft tissues is commonly called a wound. A wound is closed when the damage to the soft tissues is under the skin's surface, like a bruise. A bruise indicates bleeding under the skin. A wound is open when

the skin's surface is broken. Scrapes, cuts and punctures are open wounds. Avulsions are open wounds in which a piece of skin, soft tissue or even part of the body, such as a finger, is torn loose or is torn off entirely.

Bleeding occurs when a blood vessel is torn. With any open wound, bleeding can be severe enough to be life threatening. With an open wound, the blood comes through a tear in the skin.

Fortunately, most of the bleeding you will encounter will not be serious. It usually stops by itself within a few minutes. The blood at the wound clots and stops flowing. Sometimes, however, the

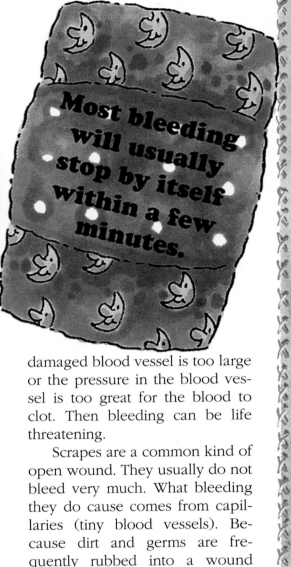

Most bleeding will usually stop by itself within a few minutes.

damaged blood vessel is too large or the pressure in the blood vessel is too great for the blood to clot. Then bleeding can be life threatening.

Scrapes are a common kind of open wound. They usually do not bleed very much. What bleeding they do cause comes from capillaries (tiny blood vessels). Because dirt and germs are frequently rubbed into a wound when a scrape occurs, it is important to clean scrapes thoroughly to prevent infection.

Punctures are usually caused by a pointed object, such as a nail, piercing the skin. If the object remains in the wound, it is called an embedded object. In most cases the object should not be removed. However, a splinter is an example of an embedded object that you can usually remove with tweezers if it is in the skin.

# A Stitch in Time

It can be difficult to judge when a wound should receive stitches from a doctor. One rule of thumb is that stitches are needed when edges of skin do not fall together or when any wound is over an inch long. Stitches speed the healing process, lessen the chances of infection and improve the appearance of scars. They should be placed within the first few hours after the injury. The following major injuries often require stitches:

- Bleeding from an artery or uncontrolled bleeding
- Wounds that show muscle or bone, involve joints, gape widely, or involve hands or feet
- Large or deep puncture wounds
- Large or deeply embedded objects
- Human or animal bites
- Wounds that, if left unattended, could leave conspicuous scars, such as those on the face

If you are caring for a wound and think it may need stitches, it probably does. Once applied, stitches are easily cared for by dabbing them with hydrogen peroxide once or twice daily. If the wound gets red or swollen or if pus begins to form, notify your health-care provider.

Stitches in the face are often removed in less than a week. In joints, they are often removed after 2 weeks. Stitches on most other body parts require removal in 6 to 10 days. Some stitches dissolve naturally and do not require removal.

# TYPES OF WOUNDS

## BRUISE
### (Contusion)
Damage to soft tissues and blood vessels causes bleeding under the skin. Tissues discolor and swell. At first, the area may only appear red. Over time, it may turn dark red or purple. A large or painful bruise may be a signal of severe damage to deep tissues.

## SCRAPE
### (Abrasion; Road rash; Rug burn; Strawberry)
Most common type of wound. Caused by skin that has been rubbed or scraped away. Usually painful because scraping away of outer layer of skin exposes nerve endings. Dirt and other matter can easily become ground into the wound, making it especially important to clean it. Can easily become infected if not kept clean.

## CUT
### (Incision; Laceration)

A cut may have either jagged or smooth edges. Cuts are commonly caused by sharp-edged objects, such as knives, scissors or broken glass. They can also result when a blow from a blunt object splits the skin. Deep cuts can damage nerves, large blood vessels and other soft tissues. Cuts usually bleed freely. Deep cuts can bleed severely. A cut may not be painful if nerves are injured.

## AVULSION

A cut in which a portion of skin or other soft tissue is partially or completely torn away. A partially avulsed piece of skin may remain but hangs like a flap. A violent force may completely tear away a body part, such as a finger. Because an avulsion often damages deeper tissues, bleeding is often significant. In contrast, when a body part is completely torn away, bleeding is easier to control because the tissues close around the vessels at the injury site.

## PUNCTURE

A wound caused when a pointed object, such as a nail, piece of glass or knife, pierces the skin. A gunshot wound is also a puncture wound. Because puncture wounds do not usually bleed a lot, they can easily become infected. Bleeding can be severe if the penetrating object damages major blood vessels or internal organs.

An object that remains embedded in the wound is called an impaled object. An object that passes completely through a body part will make two wounds—one at the entry point and one at the exit point.

# Infection

**W**hen an injury breaks the skin, the best initial defense against infection is to clean the area. For minor wounds, wash the area with soap and water. Most soaps are effective in removing harmful bacteria. You do not need to wash wounds that require medical attention because they involve more extensive tissue damage or bleeding. It is more important to control the bleeding.

Because infected wounds can cause serious medical problems, it is important to maintain an up-to-date record of immunizations. These immunizations help your body fight infection. One of these immunizations prevents tetanus, a serious disease. The best way to prevent tetanus is to receive a booster shot from your health-care provider every 10 years since the protective effect of the vaccine decreases over time.

Sometimes, even the best care for a soft tissue injury is not enough to prevent infection. You will usually be able to recognize the early signals of infection. The area around the wound becomes swollen and red. The area may feel warm or throb with pain. Some wounds discharge pus. Serious infections may cause a person to develop a fever and feel ill. Red streaks may develop that progress from the wound in the direction of the heart.

If you see any of these signals of infections, care for the wound by keeping the area clean, soaking it in warm water, elevating the affected area and applying an antibiotic ointment. Change coverings over the wound daily. If fever or red streaks develop, the infection is getting worse. If the infection persists or worsens, seek medical help.

**An infected wound may become swollen and may have a pus discharge.**

Punctures usually do not bleed very much unless a blood vessel has been injured. However, an object that goes into the soft tissues beneath the skin can carry germs deep into the body. These germs can cause infections, sometimes serious ones.

One severe infection that can result from a puncture or a deep cut is called tetanus. We all need to have the shot that protects us against tetanus and a booster shot at least every 10 years. Anyone whose skin is punctured or who is cut by an object that can carry infection, such as a rusty nail, or is bitten by an animal should check with his or her health-care provider to learn whether a booster shot is needed.

## DRESSINGS AND BANDAGES

Open wounds need some type of covering to help control bleeding and prevent infection. These coverings are often called dressings and bandages. You can buy them at drugstores and many supermarkets. You should keep assorted sizes and shapes of dressings and bandages in your first aid kit.

**Dressings are clean or sterile pads placed directly on the wound. They come in various sizes. Some have surfaces that won't stick to a wound.**

Dressings are pads placed directly on the wound to soak up blood and help keep germs out. A dressing should be sterile (free from germs). Most dressings you buy are loosely woven to let air reach the wound. This helps the wound heal. Cotton gauze dressings 2 to 4 inches square are common. Some dressings have surfaces that will not stick to a wound.

A bandage is any material used to wrap or cover any part of the body. Bandages are often used to hold dressings in place, to apply pressure that helps control bleeding and to help support an injured part of the body.

Bandages you can buy include small adhesive compresses, triangular bandages, roller bandages and bandage compresses, and thick gauze dressings attached to gauze bandages. A triangular bandage can be folded and used to cover a wound or it can be used to hold a dressing or splint in place. It can also be opened and used as a sling to

**A bandage is any material used to wrap or cover any part of the body. It is often used to hold a dressing in place. Bandages include small adhesive bandages, triangular bandages and roller bandages made of gauze or elastic material.**

support an injured arm, shoulder or hand. Roller bandages are usually made of gauze or similar material. They come in widths from 1½ to 6 inches.

To apply a roller bandage, first raise the injured area above the level of the heart, if possible, to help slow bleeding. Secure one end of the bandage in place. Then wrap the bandage around the body part, using overlapping turns, covering the dressing and extending the bandages several inches beyond the dressing at both ends. Tie or tape the bandage in place. If possible, do not cover the fingers or toes. Check them to see if they turn pale or ashen or become cold. If they do, the bandage is too tight. Loosen it.

**A folded triangular bandage can be used to secure a splint in place (*above*). An open triangular bandage can be tied as a sling to support an injured arm (*right*).**

## ROLLER BANDAGE

A roller bandage used to control bleeding is called a pressure bandage. To apply a pressure bandage ...

**1** Start by securing the bandage over the dressing.

**2** Use overlapping turns to cover the dressing completely.

**3** Tie or tape the bandage in place.

**4** Check the fingers for warmth, color and feeling every few minutes.

When a roller bandage is used to help control bleeding, it is commonly called a pressure bandage. This is because it can be applied snugly, keeping pressure over the wound. If blood soaks through bandages, put on more dressings and bandages. Do not remove blood-soaked ones.

Roller bandages can also be elastic. They are used to keep pressure on a part of the body, such as an arm or leg. They can control swelling and give support and are commonly used on joint injuries. Like other roller bandages, these elastic bandages are also available in assorted sizes.

Although an elastic bandage is very effective, it can create problems if it is applied so tightly that it restricts blood flow. Restricted blood flow is not only painful, it can cause tissue damage.

The first step in using an elastic bandage is to select the correct size. This is determined by the area that you plan to wrap. A narrow bandage would be used to wrap a hand or wrist. A medium-width bandage would be used for an arm or ankle. A wide bandage would be used to wrap a leg.

To begin the wrap, place the end of the bandage against the

**If a victim is in severe pain or can't move a body part without hurting, he or she probably has a serious injury**

skin and use overlapping turns. Gently stretch the bandage as you continue wrapping. The wrap should cover a long body section, like an arm or a calf, beginning at the point farthest from the heart. For a joint like a knee or ankle, use figure eight turns to support the joint.

Be sure that the bandage is not too tight. Check the circulation of the limb beyond the bandage by noting changes in skin color and temperature.

# CARING FOR SOFT TISSUE INJURIES

Most closed wounds, such as bruises, do not need special medical care. You can rest and immobilize the area to cut down bleeding under the skin. Applying cold can help control pain and swelling. Always put a thin layer of cloth between the source of the cold and the victim's skin. Raising the injured part helps reduce swelling. Remember RICE:

**R**est, **I**mmobilize, **C**old, **E**levation.

# ELASTIC BANDAGE

**Elastic bandages control swelling and give support for injuries such as sprains or strains. To apply an elastic bandage ...**

**Start at the point farthest from the heart.**  **1**

**Anchor the bandage.** **2**

**Wrap the bandage using overlapping turns.** **3**

**Tape the bandage in place.**  **4**

**Check the toes for warmth, color and feeling every few minutes.**  **5**

# Blood and Disease Transmission

Disease transmission occurs when bacteria or viruses from one person enter the body of another person. If a victim has an infectious disease and is bleeding severely, there is an easy path for infection to travel. If you make contact with the victim's blood or other body fluids and you have a cut, scrape or sore, a path exists for the infection to enter your body. Contact with blood or other body fluids provides an easy route for the infection to spread.

When you take action to control bleeding, it is also important to reduce the risk of infection. A properly equipped first aid kit can help you deal with a bleeding victim. Good personal hygiene practices, such as washing hands before and immediately after giving care, can also reduce the risk of disease transmission.

To reduce the risk of infection while you give care, do the following:

- Avoid being splashed by blood.
- Place a barrier between you and the victim's blood. This can be done by wearing disposable gloves when covering the wound with a dressing.
- Cover any cuts, scrapes or skin conditions you have before giving care.
- Wash your hands immediately after providing care, even if you wore gloves. Use warm running water and soap.[52] Use a utility or restroom sink. Do not use a sink in a food preparation area.
- Avoid eating, drinking and touching your mouth, eyes or nose while providing care or before you wash your hands.
- Avoid touching objects that may have been contaminated with blood.
- Avoid handling any of your personal items, such as pens or combs, while providing care or before washing your hands.

These safety precautions can greatly reduce your risk of infection. Always give first aid in ways that protect both you and the victim from disease transmission.

Some closed wounds can be extremely serious. If a victim is in severe pain or cannot move a body part without hurting, he or she probably has a serious injury. Ask yourself if the force that caused the injury was great enough to have caused serious damage. If you think it was, call 9-1-1 or the local emergency number. The victim may be bleeding internally and need emergency medical help as soon as possible.

Help the victim rest in the most comfortable position. Keep the victim from getting chilled or overheated. Reassure and comfort the victim.

---

## SIGNALS OF INTERNAL BLEEDING

Tender, swollen, bruised or hard areas of the body, such as the abdomen

Rapid, weak pulse

Skin that feels cool or moist or looks pale or bluish

Vomiting or coughing up blood

Excessive thirst

Becoming confused, faint, drowsy or unconscious

---

A major open wound has serious tissue damage and severe bleeding. To care for a major open wound, you must act at once. Do *not* waste time washing the wound. Instead, begin by placing a dressing over the wound and applying direct pressure. If a sterile dressing is not available, use any clean cloth, such as a towel, handkerchief or sock. If the victim is able to help, have him or her apply pressure to the wound. Use your own bare hand to apply pressure only as a last resort. Always try to put a barrier between yourself and a victim's blood. Keep a pair of disposable gloves handy, either in a first aid kit or in your car.

Next, elevate the wound. If possible, raise the injured area above the level of the heart. Then, apply a bandage snugly over the dressings to keep pressure on the wound. If the bleeding is still not controlled, use a pressure point. A pressure point is a spot on the body where you can squeeze the nearby artery against the bone underneath. This can slow or stop the flow of blood to the wound.

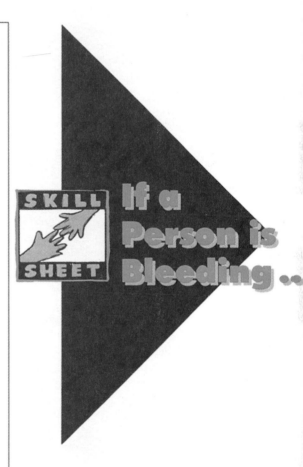

# Caring for a Major Open Wound

**Control bleeding by placing a clean covering, such as a sterile dressing, over the wound and applying pressure.**

**If you do not think the wound also involves a broken bone, elevate the injured area.**

**Apply a bandage snugly over the dressing.**

**If the bleeding cannot be controlled, put pressure on the nearby artery (pressure point).**

**Seek emergency medical attention. (Call 9-1-1 or the local emergency number.)**

**Wash your hands immediately after completing care.**

# Controlling Bleeding

**Step 1:** Check the scene and the victim.

**Step 2:** Cover the wound with a dressing and press firmly.

**Step 3:** Elevate the wound above the level of the heart.

**Step 4:** Cover the dressing with a roller bandage.

**Step 5:** If the bleeding does not stop...

Apply additional dressings.

**Step 6:** Squeeze the artery against the bone.

**Step 7:** Call, or have someone else call, 9-1-1 or the local emergency number.

**Step 8:** Care for shock.

## SHOCK

Any severe bleeding can lead to a life-threatening condition called shock. Shock is a condition in which the circulatory system fails to deliver blood to all parts of the body. When the body's organs do not receive blood, they fail to function properly. This triggers a series of responses that produce specific signals known as shock. These responses are the body's attempt to maintain adequate blood flow.

When the body is healthy, the following three conditions are needed to maintain adequate blood flow:

- The heart must be working well.
- An adequate amount of blood must be circulating in the body.
- The blood vessels must be intact and able to adjust blood flow.

When someone is injured or suddenly becomes ill, these normal body functions may be interrupted. When the injury or illness is minor, the interruption is brief because the body is able to compensate quickly. With more severe injuries or illnesses, the body may be unable to adjust. When the body is unable to meet its demands for blood, shock occurs.

Shock is likely to develop in any serious injury or illness.

## SIGNALS OF SHOCK

The signals are—

Restlessness or irritability.

Altered consciousness.

Nausea.

Pale or ashen, cool, moist skin.

Rapid breathing.

Rapid pulse.

For the heart to do its job properly, an adequate amount of blood must circulate within the body. The body can compensate for some decrease in the amount of blood. However, with severe injuries involving greater or more rapid loss of blood, the body might not be able to adjust.

# SHOCK: The Domino Effect

**A**ny serious injury or illness will trigger a series of responses in the body that act like a chain of falling dominoes. This condition is known as shock.

Shock is the body's natural attempt to keep the oxygen-rich blood flowing to the most important organs, such as the brain, heart and lungs. Without oxygen, these organs will fail to function properly. When the oxygen-deprived tissues of the arms and legs begin to die, the body sends blood back to them and away from the vital organs. As the brain is affected, the person becomes restless, drowsy and eventually becomes unconscious. As the heart is affected, it beats with an irregular pulse. The heart's rhythm becomes chaotic and the heart fails to pump blood. There is no longer a pulse. When the heart stops, breathing stops. This chain of falling dominoes eventually results in death.

# CARING FOR SHOCK

## Caring for shock involves the following simple steps:

Have the victim lie down. This is often the most comfortable position. Helping the victim rest comfortably is important because pain can intensify the body's stress and accelerate the progression of shock. Helping the victim rest in a more comfortable position may minimize any pain.

Call 9-1-1 or the local emergency number immediately. Shock cannot be managed effectively by first aid alone. A victim of shock requires emergency medical care as soon as possible.

Control any external bleeding.

Elevate the legs about 12 inches unless you suspect head, neck or back injuries or possible broken bones involving the hips or legs. If you are unsure of the victim's condition, leave him or her lying flat.

Help the victim maintain normal body temperature. If the victim is cool, try to cover him or her to avoid chilling.

Do not give the victim anything to eat or drink, even though he or she is likely to be thirsty.

Reassure the victim.

Any significant fluid loss, even as a result of diarrhea or vomiting, can cause shock. Such a decrease in body fluids affects the function of the heart. The heart eventually fails to beat properly, so the pulse becomes irregular or stops altogether.

Blood vessels act as pipelines to all parts of the body. For this circulation system to function properly, blood vessels must remain intact, preventing loss of blood. Normally, blood vessels can increase or decrease the flow of blood to different areas of the body ensuring that blood reaches the areas of the body that need it most. Injuries or illnesses, especially those that affect the brain and spinal cord, can cause blood vessels to lose this ability to regulate the flow of blood. Blood vessels can also be affected if the nervous system is damaged by infections, drugs or poisons.

If the heart is damaged, it cannot pump blood properly. If blood vessels are damaged, the body cannot adjust blood flow. Regardless of the cause, when the body does not get adequate blood, it also does not get adequate oxygen and the body goes into shock.

When shock occurs, the body attempts to adjust and send blood to the most important parts, such as the brain, heart, lungs and kidneys. The body does this by reducing blood flow to the less important parts, such as the arms, legs and skin. This is why the skin of a person in shock appears pale or ashen, especially around the lips and the eyes, and the skin feels cool.

## SPECIAL SITUATIONS

If part of the body has been torn or cut off, try to find the part and wrap it in sterile gauze or any clean material, such as a wash-cloth. Put the wrapped part in a plastic bag. Keep the part cold by placing the bag on ice, if possible, but do not freeze. Be sure the part is taken to the hospital with the victim. Doctors may be able to reattach it.

**If an object is embedded in a wound, do not remove it. Bandage bulky dressings around the object to support it in place.**

**Wrap a severed body part in sterile gauze, put it in a plastic bag and put the bag on ice. Be sure the part is taken to the hospital with the victim.**

If an object, such as a knife or a piece of glass or metal, is embedded in a wound, *do not* remove it. Place several dressings around it to keep it from moving. Bandage the dressings in place around the object. If it is only a splinter in the skin, it can be removed with tweezers. After removing the splinter from the skin, wash the area. Then cover it to keep it clean. If the splinter is in the eye, you should not attempt to remove it. Call 9-1-1 or the local emergency number; the victim needs emergency medical care.

Nose injuries are usually caused by a blow from a blunt object. The result is often a nose-bleed. High blood pressure or changes in altitude can also cause nosebleeds. In most cases, you can control bleeding by having the victim sit with the head slightly forward while pinching the nostrils together. Other meth-ods of controlling bleeding in-clude applying an ice pack to the bridge of the nose or putting pressure on the upper lip just be-neath the nose.

**To control a nosebleed, have the victim lean forward and pinch the nostrils together until bleeding stops.**

Your primary concern for injury to the mouth is to make sure the victim is able to breathe. Injuries to the mouth may cause breathing problems if blood or loose teeth obstruct the airway.

If the victim is bleeding from the mouth and you do not suspect a serious head, neck or back injury, place the victim in a seated position with the head tilted slightly forward. This will allow any blood to drain from the mouth. If this position is not possible, place the victim on his or her side in the recovery position to allow blood to drain from the mouth.

For injuries that penetrate the lip, place a rolled dressing between the lip and the gum. You can place another dressing on the outer surface of the lip. If the tongue is bleeding, apply a dressing and direct pressure. Applying cold to the lips or tongue can help reduce swelling and ease pain.

If a victim's tooth is knocked out, control the bleeding and save the tooth so it possibly can be reinserted. To control the bleeding, place the tooth in the socket or roll a sterile dressing and insert it into the space left by the missing tooth only if the victim is fully

**To control bleeding inside the cheek, place folded dressings inside the mouth against the wound *(top)*. To control bleeding on the outside, use dressings to apply pressure directly to the wound and bandage so as not to restrict breathing *(bottom)*.**

**If a tooth is knocked out, place a sterile dressing directly in the space left by the tooth. Tell the victim to bite down.**

conscious and able to cooperate. Have the victim gently bite down to maintain pressure.

For minor open wounds that do not bleed very much, such as scrapes, wash the wound thoroughly with soap and water. Put a sterile dressing over the wound and apply pressure for a few minutes, if necessary, to control any bleeding. When bleeding is controlled, take off the dressing and put an antibiotic ointment on the wound. Then cover the wound with a clean dressing and bandage.

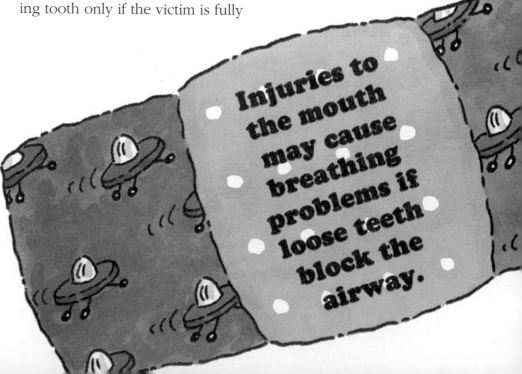

Injuries to the mouth may cause breathing problems if loose teeth block the airway.

# NOW 'SMILE!'

**K**nocked-out teeth no longer have to lead to gapped smiles and bridgework. Most dentists can successfully replant a knocked-out tooth if they can do so quickly and if the tooth has been cared for properly.

Replanting a tooth is similar to replanting a tree. On each tooth, tiny root fibers attach to the jawbone to hold the tooth in place. Inside the tooth a canal filled with bundles of blood vessels and nerves runs from the tooth and into the jawbone and surrounding tissue.

When these fibers and tissues are torn from the socket, it is important for them to be replaced within 30 minutes to an hour after injury. Generally, the sooner the tooth is replaced, the better the chance it will survive. The knocked-out tooth must be handled carefully. Pick up the victim's tooth by the chewing edge (crown), not the root. Do not rub or handle the root part of the tooth.

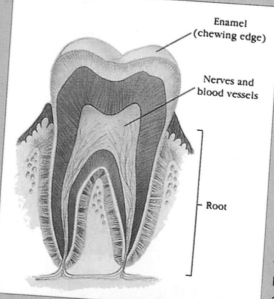

Enamel (chewing edge)

Nerves and blood vessels

Root

If the victim is willing and able to cooperate, place the tooth back in the socket in its normal position after rinsing it in milk. Have the victim bite down gently or hold the tooth in position with a sterile gauze pad, a tissue or a clean cloth or the victim can use the tongue.[53] Be sure to see your dentist as soon as possible.

If you are unable to put the tooth back in its socket, preserve the tooth by placing it in a closed container of cool, fresh milk. If milk is not available, use the victim's saliva. Do not use water. Be sure to take the container with the injured tooth to the dentist.

A dentist or emergency room physician will clean the tooth. The tooth will then be placed back in the socket and secured with a special splint. The splint will hold the tooth stable while the fibers reattach to the jawbone. The bundles of blood vessels and nerves will grow back within 6 to 8 weeks.

**A puncture wound that penetrates the lung or the chest cavity surrounding the lung allows air to go in and out of the cavity.**

Air from lung filling space around lung

Air from outside filling space around lung

BULLET PENETRATES CHEST CAVITY

jury to these areas can be life threatening. Care for any life-threatening conditions first, then give any additional care that is needed.

The chest is the upper part of the trunk, formed by the ribs, breastbone and spine. It contains the heart, lungs and muscles that control breathing. A puncture wound to the chest can range from minor to life threatening. Stab and gunshot wounds are examples of puncture injuries.

A forceful puncture to the chest may penetrate the rib cage. This could allow air to freely pass in and out of the chest through the wound. This prevents the lungs from working normally. With each breath the victim takes, you may hear a sucking sound coming from the wound. This is the main signal of a penetrating chest injury called a sucking chest wound. The penetrating object can also injure structures within the chest, including the lungs, heart or major arteries or veins.

Without care, the victim's condition will quickly get worse. One or both lungs will fail to work properly and breathing will

Most injuries to the chest and abdomen are only minor cuts, scratches and bruises. Sometimes, more serious injuries can occur, such as those resulting from motor vehicle accidents, falls, stabs and bullet wounds. These injuries can cause severe bleeding or make breathing difficult. Because the chest and abdomen hold many organs important to life, in-

**A special dressing with one loose corner keeps air from the wound when breathing in and allows air to escape when breathing out.**

BREATHING IN

BREATHING OUT

Lodged bullet

Injured lung

become more difficult. Your number one concern is the victim's breathing problem.

To care for a sucking chest wound, cover the wound with a dressing that does not allow air to pass through it. A plastic bag, a disposable glove, a piece of plastic wrap or aluminum foil folded several times and placed over the wound will work if a special sterile dressing is not available. Tape the dressing in place, except for one corner that should stay loose. If none of these materials are available, use a folded cloth. Give any other care that is necessary.

The abdomen is the soft area of the belly, below the chest. Because the abdomen is not protected by any bones, it is easily injured. A forceful blow to the abdomen or a fall from a height can cause severe bleeding inside the body. If you suspect severe internal bleeding, keep the victim lying flat and watch for signals of internal bleeding. Bending the knees and hips slightly may make the victim more comfortable. A folded blanket or a pillow can be placed under the knees to support the legs in this position. If movement of the legs causes pain, leave the victim lying flat.

Sometimes a severe blow or penetrating injury to the abdomen can cause organs to be exposed or protrude. In this case, carefully position the victim on his or her back. Do not apply any pressure to the organs and do not attempt to push the organs back inside. Remove any clothing from around the wound and apply moist, sterile dressings or a moistened clean cloth loosely over the wound. Use warm tap water to moisten the dressings.

Wounds that break through the abdomen can cause the organs to push out. Carefully remove clothing from around the wound. Cover the organs with a moist sterile or clean dressing and cover the dressing with plastic wrap. Place a folded towel or other cloth over the dressing to keep the organs warm.

# BURNS

## Burns are a specific type of soft tissue injury.

Burns caused by heat are the most common. Certain chemicals, however, can also cause burns. Electrical current can burn the body internally and externally. Radiation from the sun can cause sunburn. A burn first destroys the top layer of skin. If it continues to burn, it injures or destroys the second layer of skin. When burns break the skin, they can cause infection and loss of fluid from the body and can damage the body's ability to control its temperature.

A critical burn
can be
life threatening
and needs
immediate
medical
attention.

Deep burns can also damage the victim's ability to breathe.

The severity of a burn depends on the temperature of whatever caused the burn and the length of time the victim is exposed to it. The severity is also affected by the burn's location on the body, the size of the burn and the victim's age and medical condition.

You can describe burns by their cause—heat, electricity, chemicals and radiation—or by their depth. The deeper the burn, the more severe it is.

A burn that involves only the top layer of skin is the least severe. The skin is red and dry and the burn hurts. These burns usually heal in 5 to 6 days and do not leave scars.

Deeper burns are also red. They have blisters that may open and seep clear fluid. The burned skin may look blotchy. These burns are usually painful and the area often swells.

Some burns destroy all the layers of skin and the tissues underneath. They can even destroy bones. These burns look brown or blackish. The tissues underneath may appear white. These burns can sometimes be surprisingly pain-free because nerve endings have been destroyed. These burns are critical.

A critical burn needs immediate medical attention. Critical burns can be life threatening. It is not always easy to tell how severe a burn is right after it has happened. Call 9-1-1 or the local emergency number if a burn victim is having trouble breathing or has burns on more than one part of the body. Also call if the victim has burns on the head, neck, hands, feet or genitals. Call for any burns caused by chemicals, explosions or electricity.

Burns caused by flames or hot grease usually need medical attention, especially if the victim is

# Critical Burns

Burns involving trouble breathing

Burns covering more than one body part

Burns to the head, neck, hands, feet or genitals

Burns (other than a very minor one) to a child
or an elderly person

Burns resulting from chemicals,
explosions or electricity

a child or elderly. Burns caused by hot liquid or flames that contact clothing also are serious, since the clothing keeps the heat in contact with the skin. Some fabrics even melt and stick to the skin. All these burns may look minor at first but they can continue to get worse.

## CARE FOR BURNS

To care for a burn, follow these basic steps. First, stop the burning. For example, you may have to put out flames that have caught clothing. Remove all rings, watches, jewelry and belts since they can retain heat and cause a tourniquet-like effect because of changes in the body tissues.[54] Next, use water to cool the burned area. Do not use ice except on minor burns, such as a burned finger from touching a hot stove.

After cooling the burned area for several minutes, cover the burn with a dry, clean dressing to help prevent infection. Bandage loosely—do not put any pressure on the burn. Do not put any kind of ointment on a burn unless it is a very minor burn. Ointment may seal in heat and does not do much to relieve pain. Do not use other home remedies like butter or grease; they can cause infection. Do not break blisters; keeping the skin unbroken helps prevent infection.

For minor burns and burns with open blisters that are not bad enough to need medical care, wash the area with soap and water. Keep it clean. Put on an antibiotic ointment. Watch for signals of infection.

Have the victim of severe burns lie down unless he or she is having trouble breathing. Do not remove clothing if it is stuck to the burned skin. Raise burned areas above the level of the heart, if possible. Burn victims chill easily, so protect the victim from drafts and keep the victim dry.

## SPECIAL KINDS OF BURNS

Chemical burns can happen both in the workplace and at home. Certain chemicals used in laboratory work and other jobs can cause severe burns if they

**To care for a burn, first stop the burning.**

**Cool the burned area with large amounts of cool water.**

**Then cover the burn with dry, clean or sterile dressings to help prevent infection.**

## Superficial Burn

**(First Degree)**

Involves only the top layer of skin. The skin is red and dry and the burn is usually painful. The area may swell. Most sunburns are superficial burns. Superficial burns usually heal in 5 to 6 days without permanent scarring.

## Partial Thickness Burn

**(Second Degree)**

Involves the top layers of skin. The skin is red and has blisters that may open and seep clear fluid, making the skin appear wet. The burned skin may appear mottled. These burns are usually painful and the area often swells. The burn usually heals in 3 to 4 weeks. Scarring may occur.

## Full Thickness Burn

**(Third Degree)**

Destroys all layers of skin and any or all of the underlying structures—fat, muscles, bones and nerves. These burns look brown or black (charred) with the tissues underneath sometimes appearing white. They can either be extremely painful or relatively painless if the burn destroys the nerve endings.

# CARE FOR BURNS

The care for burns involves the following four basic steps:

**1** **Stop the Burning.**
Put out flames or remove the victim from the source of the burn.

**2** *Call Fast.*
For a serious burn, have someone else call 9-1-1 or the local emergency number while you provide care. If you are alone, provide 1 minute of care, then make the call.

**3** **Cool the Burn.**
Use large amounts of cool water to cool the burned area. Do not use ice or ice water other than on small superficial burns. Ice causes body heat loss. Use whatever resources are available—tub, shower or garden hose, for example. You can apply soaked towels, sheets or other wet cloths to a burned face or other areas that cannot be immersed. Be sure to keep the cloths cool by adding more water.

**4** **Cover the Burn.**
Use dry, sterile dressings or a clean cloth. Loosely bandage them in place. Covering the burn helps keep out air and reduces pain. Covering the burn also helps prevent infection. If the burn covers a large area of the body, cover it with clean, dry sheets or other cloth.

# Within Striking Distance

In medieval times, people believed that ringing church bells would get rid of lightning during thunderstorms. It was an unfortunate superstition for bell ringers. In 33 years, lightning struck 386 church steeples and 103 bell ringers died.[55]

Church bell ringers have dropped off the list of people most likely to be struck during a thunderstorm, but lightning strikes remain very dangerous. The National Center for Injury Prevention and Control reports that during the last 40 years, about 90 people have died each year after being struck by lightning in the United States.[56] In general, the greatest number of deaths were reported during June and August, followed by July and May.

Lightning occurs when particles of water, ice and air moving inside storm clouds lose electrons. Eventually, the cloud becomes divided into layers of positive and negative particles. Most electrical current remains inside the cloud. Sometimes, however, the negative charge flashes toward the ground, which has a positive charge. An electrical current snakes back and forth between the cloud and the ground many times in the seconds that we see a flash crackle down from the sky. Anything tall— a tower, a tree or a person— becomes a path for the electrical current.

Traveling at speeds up to 300 miles per second, a lightning strike can hurl a person through the air. It can burn clothes off and can sometimes cause the heart to stop beating. The most severe lightning strikes carry up to 50 million volts of electricity, enough to serve 13,000 homes. Lightning can "flash" over a person's body or it can travel through blood vessels and nerves to reach the ground.

Besides burns, lightning can also cause nervous system damage, broken bones and loss of hearing or eyesight. Victims sometimes act confused and suffer memory loss. They may describe what happened as getting hit on the head or hearing an explosion.

Use common sense during thunderstorms. If you see a storm approaching in the distance, don't wait until you are soaked to seek shelter. If a thunderstorm threatens,[57] you should—

◆ Go inside a large building or home with four solid walls and preferably with electrical, telephone and plumbing lines, which aid in grounding the structure.
◆ Go inside a car and roll up the windows. Do not touch any of the car's metal framework when in the car.
◆ Stop swimming or boating as soon as you see or hear a storm since water conducts electricity.
◆ Stay away from the telephone, except in an emergency.
◆ Do not shower or bathe during a thunderstorm.
◆ Stay away from telephone poles and tall trees if you are caught outside.
◆ Stay off hilltops; try to crouch down in a ravine or valley.
◆ Stay away from farm equipment and small metal vehicles, such as motorcycles, bicycles and golf carts.
◆ Avoid wire fences, wire clotheslines, some fishing rods, metal pipes and rails and other conductors.
◆ Stay several yards apart if you are in a group.

contact the skin or eyes; so can various household products, such as cleansers, lawn and garden sprays, paint removers and household bleach. The stronger the chemical and the longer the contact, the worse the burn. The chemical continues to burn as long as it is on the skin. You must remove the chemical from the skin as quickly as possible and call 9-1-1 or the local emergency number. If possible, have someone call while you care for the victim.

For liquid chemical burns to the skin or eyes, flush the burn with large amounts of cool running water until EMS personnel arrive and take over. Have the victim take off any clothes with the chemical on them, if possible. If only one eye has been exposed to the chemical, flush the affected eye from the nose outward to prevent washing the chemical into the unaffected eye.

**In general, flush a liquid chemical burn to the skin (top) or eyes (bottom) with cool running water until EMS arrives.**

Flush a chemical burn to the skin or eyes with large amounts of cool running water.

---

# DOs & DON'Ts OF BURN CARE [58]

### DOs

Do cool a burn by flushing with water.

Do cover the burn with a dry, clean covering, such as a sterile dressing.

Do keep the victim comfortable.

Do keep the victim from getting chilled or overheated.

### DON'Ts

Don't apply ice directly to any burn unless it is very minor.

Don't touch a burn with anything except a clean covering.

Don't remove pieces of cloth that stick to the burned area.

Don't try to clean a severe burn.

Don't break blisters.

Don't use any kind of ointment on a severe burn.

An electrical burn may severely damage underlying tissues.

Never go near a victim you think has been injured by electricity until you are sure the power has been turned off.

For dry chemical burns, dust off as much as possible with gloved hands, a brush or towel.

Electrical burns can happen at home, at work or wherever a person comes in contact with electricity. Sources of electricity include power lines, lightning, defective electrical household equipment and unprotected electrical outlets. Coming in contact with one of these sources can send electricity through the body. The severity of a burn depends on how long the body is in contact with the electric current, the strength of the current, the type of current and the direction it takes through the body. These burns are often deep. The victim may have two wounds, one where the current entered the body and one where it left. Although these wounds may look minor, the tissues beneath them may be severely damaged.

Never go near a victim whom you think has been injured by electricity until you are sure the power is turned off. *If a power line is down, wait for the fire department or the power company.* If there are people in a car with a downed wire across or under it, tell them not to move and to stay in the car.

With an electrical burn, the burn itself will not be the major problem. Check breathing and signs of circulation if the victim is unconscious. Check for other injuries, such as possible fractures. The victim may have a head, neck or back injury, so do not move him or her. Cover an electrical burn with a dry, sterile dressing. Because of the danger of possible electrocution and the likelihood that the burn is deep and involves damaged nerves that do not feel pain, do not cool the burn with water. Keep the victim from getting chilled.

Radiation from the sun and other sources can cause painful burns that may blister. Cool the burn. A doctor or pharmacist can tell you about products to put on mild burns such as a minor sunburn. The victim can protect the burn from further damage by staying out of the sun. If you are going to be spending time in direct sun, it is wise to wear a protective lotion or cream.

People are unlikely to be exposed to other types of radiation unless they work in special settings. If they do, they are trained to prevent exposure.

Most of the burns you will have to deal with will be minor ones. Cool them, put on an antibiotic ointment and cover them to prevent infection. If you encounter a victim with a more severe burn, stop the burning and cover the burned area to prevent infection. Keep the victim from getting chilled and call 9-1-1 or your local emergency number. If the burn was caused by electricity, check for life-threatening conditions and other complications, such as fractures. Cover the burned area with a dry dressing. If the victim was burned by a liquid chemical, flush the burn with water until EMS personnel arrive and take over.

Solar radiation burns can be painful.

# TOO MUCH OF A GOOD THING

Contrary to some beliefs, tan is not in. Although brief exposure to the sun causes your skin to produce the vitamin D necessary for the healthy formation of bones, long exposure can cause problems, such as sunburn, skin cancer and early aging—a classic case of too much of a good thing being bad. According to the American Academy of Dermatology, there is no known safe way to tan because there is no "safe" UV light.[59]

There are two kinds of ultraviolet (UV) light rays to be concerned about. Ultraviolet beta rays (UVB) are the burn-producing rays that more commonly cause skin cancer. These are the rays that damage the skin's surface and cause you to blister and peel. The other rays, ultraviolet alpha rays (UVA), have been heralded by tanning salons as "safe rays." Although UVA rays may not appear as harmful as UVB rays to the skin's surface, they more readily penetrate the deeper layers of the skin. This increases the risk of skin cancer, skin aging, eye damage and changes that may alter the skin's ability to fight disease.

How do you get enough sun without getting too much? First, avoid exposure to the sun between 10:00 a.m. and 4:00 p.m. UV rays are most harmful during this period. Second, wear proper clothing, which includes a shirt that covers the shoulders and a hat that shades the head, back of the neck, face and eyes. Third, if you are going to be exposed to the sun, protect your skin and eyes.

Commercial sunscreens come in various strengths. The

American Academy of Dermatology recommends year-round sun protection including use of a sunscreen with a Sun Protection Factor (SPF) of 15 or greater for everyone, but particularly for people who are fair-skinned and sunburn easily. Apply sunscreen 15 to 30 minutes before exposure to the sun and reapply it often (every 60 to 90 minutes). Swimmers should use sunscreens labeled as water-resistant and reapply them as described on the label. Do not forget to apply lip balm that contains sunscreen with an SPF of 15 or greater.

Your best bet is to use a sunscreen that claims to protect against both UVB and UVA rays. Carefully check the label to determine the protection a product offers. Some products only offer protection against UVB rays.

It is equally important to protect your eyes from sun damage. Sunglasses are a sunscreen for your eyes and provide important protection from UV rays. Be sure to wear sunglasses that are labeled with their UV-absorbing ability. Ophthalmologists recommend sunglasses that have a UV absorption of 99-100 percent.[60] Darker lenses are not necessarily better; the UV protection comes from application of a chemical coating, not the lens color.

The next time the sun beckons, put on a shirt, hat, some sunscreen and your sunglasses. Then, go outside and have a great time.

It's a beautiful, sunny Saturday afternoon, and where are you? In the hospital emergency room, that's where, with a knee hurting so bad you had to borrow crutches to get there. Maybe it's time to give up the weekend athletics. You pass the time waiting your turn and watching other visitors. They come in all ages and sizes. Here's a 14-year-old football player complete with anxious parents and

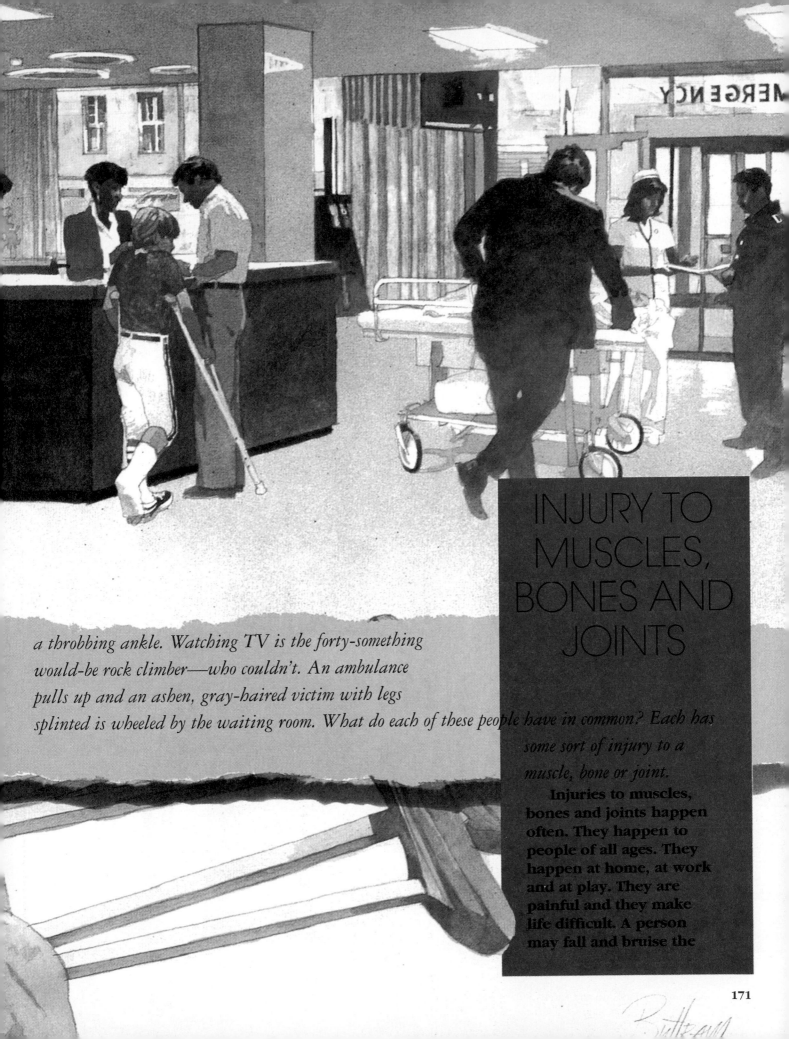

a throbbing ankle. Watching TV is the forty-something would-be rock climber—who couldn't. An ambulance pulls up and an ashen, gray-haired victim with legs splinted is wheeled by the waiting room. What do each of these people have in common? Each has some sort of injury to a muscle, bone or joint.

# INJURY TO MUSCLES, BONES AND JOINTS

Injuries to muscles, bones and joints happen often. They happen to people of all ages. They happen at home, at work and at play. They are painful and they make life difficult. A person may fall and bruise the muscles of one leg, making walking painful. Equipment may fall on a worker and break bones. A person bracing one hand against the dashboard in an automobile accident may injure the bones at the shoulder and disable the arm. A skier may fall and twist a leg, tearing muscles and making it impossible to stand or move.

Injuries like these are almost always painful, but they are rarely life threatening. If they are not recognized and cared for, how-ever, they can cause serious problems and even disable the victim.

The body's skeleton is made up of bones and muscles and the tendons and ligaments that connect them. Together, they give the body shape and stability. Bones and muscles connect to form various parts of the body. They work together to allow the body to move.

Muscles are soft tissues. The body has over 600 muscles, most of them attached to bones by strong tissues called tendons. Un-like other soft tissues, muscles are able to shorten and lengthen—contract and relax. This contracting and relaxing is what makes the body move. The brain directs the muscles to move through the spinal cord, a pathway of nerves in the spine. Tiny jolts of electricity called electrical impulses travel through the nerves to the muscles. They cause the muscles to contract. When the muscles contract, they pull at the bones, causing motion at a joint.

# MUSCLES

**The body has over 600 muscles, most of them attached to bones by strong tissues called tendons. The shortening and lengthening of the muscles is what makes the body move.**

**FRONT VIEW**

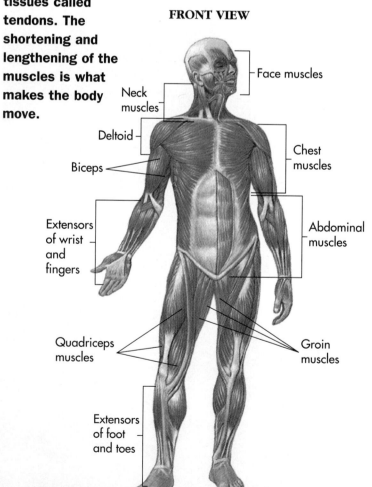

Face muscles
Neck muscles
Deltoid
Biceps
Chest muscles
Extensors of wrist and fingers
Abdominal muscles
Quadriceps muscles
Groin muscles
Extensors of foot and toes

**BACK VIEW**

Neck muscles
Back muscles
Deltoid
Triceps
Extensors of wrist and fingers
Gluteus maximus
Hamstring muscles
Calf muscles
Achilles tendon

Injuries to the brain, the spinal cord or the nerves can affect muscle control. When nerves lose control of muscles, it is called paralysis. When a muscle is injured, a nearby muscle often takes over for the injured one.

Approximately 200 bones in various sizes and shapes form the skeleton. The skeleton protects many of the organs inside the body. Bones are hard and dense. Because they are strong and rigid, they are not injured easily. Bones

To brain

Brain

Connecting nerve cell

Motor nerve

Spinal cord

Sensory nerve

**Messages are sent to and from the brain by way of nerves.**

# BONES

**Over 200 bones in various sizes and shapes form the skeleton. The skeleton protects many of the organs inside the body.**

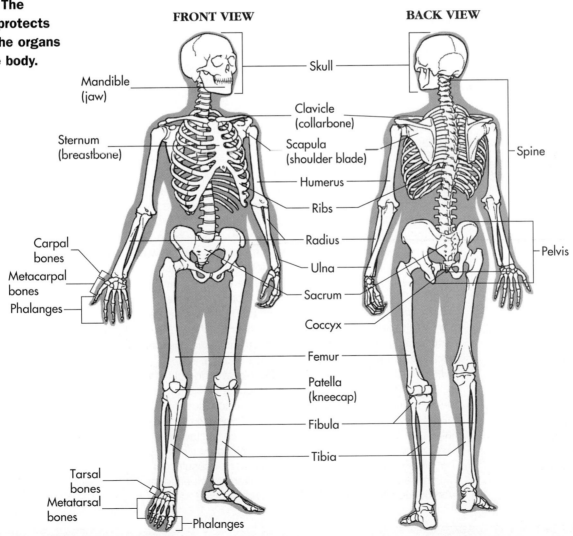

**FRONT VIEW**

**BACK VIEW**

Skull

Mandible (jaw)

Clavicle (collarbone)

Sternum (breastbone)

Scapula (shoulder blade)

Spine

Humerus

Ribs

Carpal bones

Radius

Metacarpal bones

Ulna

Pelvis

Phalanges

Sacrum

Coccyx

Femur

Patella (kneecap)

Fibula

Tibia

Tarsal bones

Metatarsal bones

Phalanges

# The Breaking Point

Osteoporosis is a bone disorder that is a "silent" disease going on for decades before a person experiences symptoms, usually after reaching the age of 60. Twenty eight million Americans have osteoporosis; 80 percent of those affected are women.[61] Fair-skinned women with ancestors from northern Europe, the British Isles, Japan or China are most likely to develop osteoporosis. One and a half million spine, hip, wrist and other fractures occur annually in the U.S. because of osteoporosis.[62] An American woman's risk of hip fracture alone is equal to her combined risk of breast, uterine and ovarian cancer.

Osteoporosis occurs when the calcium content of bone decreases. Normal bones are hard, dense tissues that endure great stresses. Calcium is a key to bone growth, development and repair. When the calcium content of bones decreases, bones become frail and less dense. They are less able to repair the normal damage they incur. This leaves bones, especially hips, back and wrists, more prone to fractures. These fractures may occur with only a little force. Some even occur without force.

The victim may be taking a walk or washing dishes when the fracture occurs.

Osteoporosis can begin as early as age 30. The amount of calcium a person absorbs from his or her diet declines with age, making calcium intake more important as you get older.

Building strong bones before age 35 is the key to preventing osteoporosis. Calcium and exercise are necessary to bone building. Three to four daily servings of low-fat dairy products should provide enough calcium. Vitamin D also is necessary because it helps the body to absorb calcium to form strong bones. Exposure to sunshine enables the body to make vitamin D. Dark-skinned and elderly people need more exposure to the sun. People who do not receive adequate exposure to the sun need to eat foods that contain vitamin D. The best sources are vitamin-fortified milk and fatty fish, such as tuna, salmon and eel.

People who do not take in adequate calcium can obtain calcium supplements. Some are combined with vitamin D. However, before taking a calcium supplement, consult your health-care provider. Many highly advertised calcium supplements are ineffective because they do not dissolve in the body.

Weight-bearing exercise increases bone density and the activity of bone-building cells. Regular exercise may reduce the rate of bone loss by promoting new bone formation. It may also stimulate the skeletal system to repair itself. An effective exercise program, such as aerobics, jogging or walking, involves the weight-bearing bones and muscles of the legs.

If you have any questions about your health and osteoporosis, consult your health-care provider. Take care of your bones and do not let osteoporosis get you down.

have a rich supply of blood and nerves. Bone injuries can bleed and they usually hurt. If the injury is not cared for, the bleeding can become life threatening. Bones weaken with age. Children have more flexible bones than adults; their bones break less easily. Older adults have more brittle bones. Sometimes they break surprisingly easily. This gradual weakening of bones is called osteoporosis.

The ends of two or more bones coming together at one place form a joint. The bones at a joint are held together by strong, tough bands called ligaments. All joints have a normal range of movement—an area in which they can move freely without too much stress or strain. When joints are forced beyond this range, ligaments stretch and tear.

The four basic types of injuries to muscles, bones and joints are fractures, dislocations, strains and sprains. They happen in a variety of ways. A fracture is either a complete break, a chip or a crack in a bone. It can be caused by a fall, a blow and sometimes

**Fractures include chipped or cracked bones and bones broken all the way through the skin.**

even a twisting movement. Fractures are open or closed. An open fracture involves an open wound. It occurs when an arm or a leg bends in such a way that bone ends tear through the skin. An object that goes into the skin and

breaks the bone, such as a bullet, can also cause an open fracture. In a closed fracture the skin is not broken. Closed fractures are more common. Open fractures are more dangerous; they carry a risk of infection and severe bleeding. In general, fractures are life threatening only if they involve breaks in large bones such as the thigh, sever an artery or affect breathing. Since you cannot always tell if a person has a fracture, you should consider the cause of the injury. A fall from a height or a motor vehicle accident, for instance, could signal a possible fracture.

Dislocations are usually more obvious than fractures. A dislocation is the movement of a bone at a joint away from its normal position. This movement is usually caused by a violent force tearing the ligaments that hold the bones in place. When a bone is moved out of place, the joint no longer

**A typical joint consists of two or more bones held together by ligaments.**

THE KNEE

Femur

Ligaments

Ligaments

Tibia

Fibula

Tendon

Patella

functions. The displaced bone end often forms a bump, a ridge or a hollow that does not normally exist.

A sprain is the tearing of ligaments at a joint. Mild sprains may swell but usually heal quickly. The victim might not feel much pain and is active again soon. If a victim ignores the signals of swelling and pain and becomes active too soon, the joint will not heal properly and will remain weak. There is a good chance it will become reinjured, only this time more severely. A severe sprain can also involve a fracture or dislocation of the bones at the joint. The joints most easily injured are at the ankle, knee, wrist and fingers.

A strain is a stretching and tearing of muscles or tendons. Strains are often caused by lifting something heavy or working a muscle too hard. They usually involve the muscles in the neck, back, thigh or the back of the lower leg. Some strains can reoccur, especially in the neck and back.

**A dislocation is a separation of a bone from its position at a joint.**

How can you tell how bad the injury is to a muscle, bone or joint? Often you cannot. Sometimes an X-ray, Computer Aided Tomography (CAT scan) or Magnetic Resonance Imaging (MRI) is needed to determine the extent of the injury. Certain signals, however, can give you a clue regarding whether the injury is severe.

One of the most common signals is pain. The injured area may

## Signals of Serious Muscle, Bone or Joint Injuries

Always suspect a serious injury when the following signals are present:

Significant deformity.

Bruising and swelling.

Inability to use the affected part normally.

Bone fragments sticking out of a wound.

Victim feels bones grating; victim felt or heard a snap or pop at the time of injury.

The injured area is cold and numb.

Cause of the injury suggests that the injury may be severe.

COSF-Boston

**Serious bone or joint injuries may appear deformed.**

# SPRAINS VERSUS STRAINS

**W**hether an injury is a sprain or strain is often confusing. A sprain is the partial or complete stretching or tearing of the special soft tissue bands that hold bones together at a joint, called ligaments. A strain is a stretching or tearing of muscles or the strong fibers that attach muscle to bone, called tendons. In short, injuries to joints are usually sprains; injuries to the soft tissue between joints, the muscles and tendons, are strains.

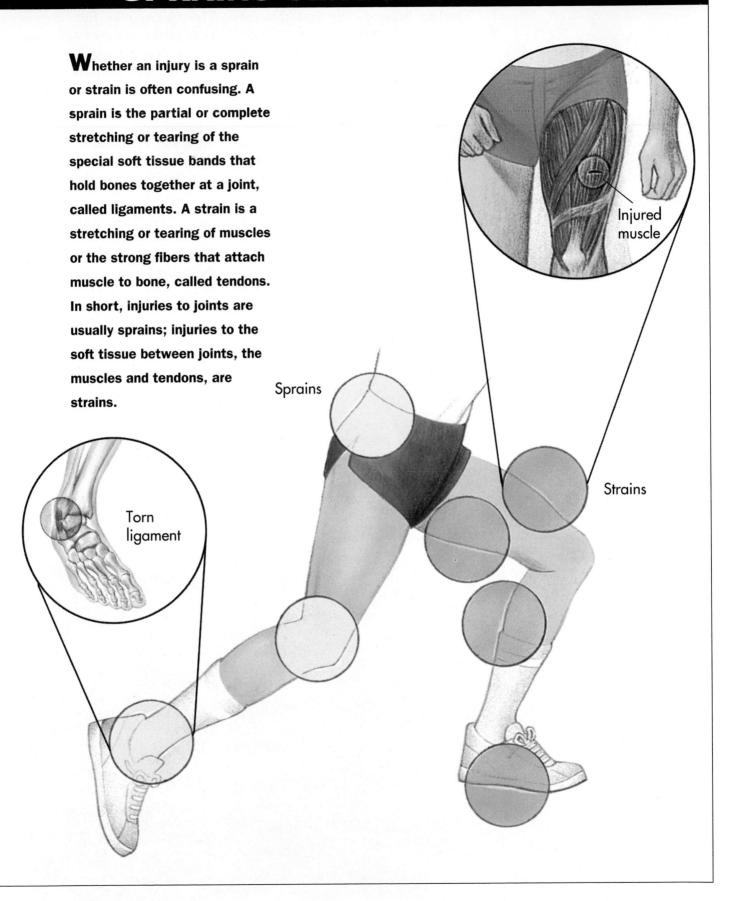

Injured muscle

Sprains

Strains

Torn ligament

IF YOU SUSPECT
A SERIOUS
MUSCLE, BONE OR
JOINT INJURY, YOU
MUST KEEP THE
INJURED PART FROM
MOVING.

be painful to touch and to move. The area may be swollen and red or bruised. The area may be twisted or strangely bent. It may have abnormal lumps, ridges and hollows.

A good way to tell if an area is not normal is to compare it with an uninjured part. For example, if you compare an arm you think may be fractured or dislocated with the uninjured one, you may be able to spot something that looks strange or out of place. The victim may hear a snap or pop at the time of the injury or feel bones grating. Hands and fingers or feet and toes may feel numb or tingly.

When caring for a muscle, bone or joint injury, always check and care for life-threatening conditions first, even if the victim is in pain. Then check for other in-

**To immobilize a bone, a splint must include the joints above and below the fracture.**

**To immobilize a joint, a splint must include the bones above and below the injured joint.**

# Splinting

**S**plint only if the victim must be moved or transported by someone other than emergency medical personnel.

**S**plint only if you can do it without causing more pain and discomfort to the victim.

**S**plint an injury in the position you find it.

**S**plint the injured area and the joints above and below the injury.

**C**heck for proper circulation before and after splinting.

juries. If you find what appears to be an injury to a muscle, bone or joint, you must decide whether to call 9-1-1 or the local emergency number.

Call 9-1-1 or the local emergency number if the victim's head, neck or back is injured, if the victim has any trouble breathing or if the victim is unable to move or use the injured part without pain. If you think the victim might have a head, neck or back injury, leave the victim lying flat.

You do not need to know what kind of injury it is to care for it. Proper care includes making the victim more comfortable. You can apply ice to control swelling and help reduce pain. Most important, minimize movement of the injured part. This can be done by helping to support it with something such as a pillow. Be careful not to move the victim in any way that causes pain.

If you are going to move or transport the victim, you must immobilize the injured part. One way to do this is to splint it. Splint only if you can do it without hurting the victim. Attempt to splint an injury in the position in which you find it. Splint the injured area and the joints above and below the area. Check for circulation before and after splinting to make sure the splint is not too tight.

There are a variety of ways you can immobilize an injured body part. One method is to use the victim's body to splint an injured area. For example, you can splint an arm to the chest or an injured leg to the uninjured leg. A part of the body used as a splint is called an anatomic splint.

**A part of the body used as a splint is called an anatomic splint. For instance, an injured leg can be splinted to the uninjured leg.**

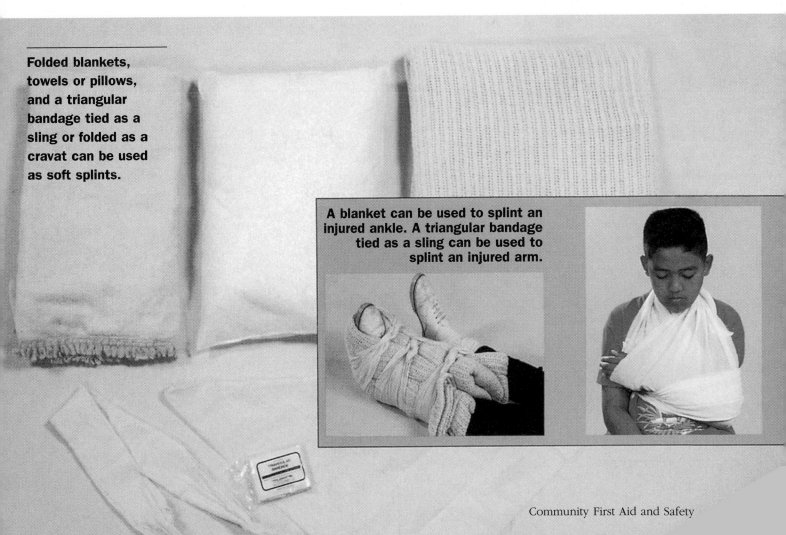

**Folded blankets, towels or pillows, and a triangular bandage tied as a sling or folded as a cravat can be used as soft splints.**

**A blanket can be used to splint an injured ankle. A triangular bandage tied as a sling can be used to splint an injured arm.**

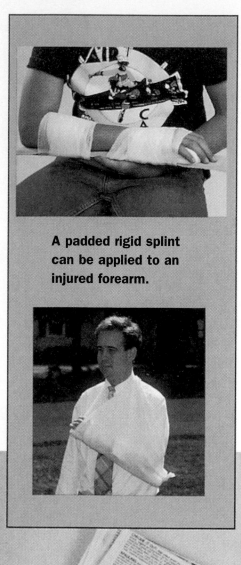

A padded rigid splint can be applied to an injured forearm.

You can make a soft splint from soft materials such as a folded blanket, towels or pillows. A soft splint can also be made from a folded triangular bandage. A sling, another kind of soft splint, is a triangular bandage tied to support an injured arm, wrist or hand. You can also use rigid splints such as boards, folded magazines and newspapers or metal strips (that do not have any sharp edges) to immobilize the injury.

Remember, the purpose of splinting is to keep an injured part from moving. If a victim with an injured leg is sitting or lying so that the leg is stretched out on the ground, the ground will work as a splint.

After you have splinted the injury, apply ice and elevate the injured part. Keep the victim from getting chilled or overheated and be reassuring. Some injuries, such as a broken finger, do not require you to call 9-1-1 or the local emergency number but still need medical attention. When transporting the victim, have someone else drive, if possible, so you can keep an eye on the victim and give any necessary care.

General care for all musculoskeletal injuries is similar. Remember rest, immobilize, cold and elevation (R.I.C.E.).

Boards, folded newspapers and magazines can be used as rigid splints.

# Sprains and Strains

**S**pring is the season of flowers, trees, strains and sprains. Almost as soon as armchair athletes come out of hibernation to become intramural heroes, emergency clinics see an increase in sprained ankles, twisted knees and strained backs. So what do you do when you attempt the first slide of the softball season and wind up injured?

When a person twists an ankle or strains his or her back, the tissues underneath the skin are injured. Blood and fluids seep from the torn blood vessels and cause swelling to occur at the site of the injury. By keeping the injured area cool, you can help control internal bleeding and reduce pain. Cold causes the broken blood vessels to constrict, limiting the blood and fluids that seep out. Cold also reduces muscle spasms and numbs the nerve endings. Never put ice directly on bare skin. Ice should be applied to the injury periodically for about 48-72 hours or until the swelling goes away. If pain persists beyond 2-3 days and you have not already done so, be sure to see your health-care provider as soon as possible.

If a Person is Unable to Move or Use an Injured Part ...

**STRAIN**

**SPRAIN**

An injury causes damage to blood vessels, causing bleeding in the injured area. Injury irritates nerve endings, causing pain.

Applying ice or a cold pack constricts blood vessels, slowing bleeding that causes the injury to swell. Cold deadens the nerve endings, relieving pain.

Applying heat dialates blood vessels, increasing blood flow to the injured area. Nerve endings become more sensitive.

# Apply a Soft Splint

**Step 1:** Check the scene and the victim.

**Step 2:** Support the injured area above and below the site of the injury.

**Step 3:** Check for feeling, warmth and color.

**Step 4:** Place several folded triangular bandages above and below the injured area.

**Step 5:** Tie triangular bandages securely.

**Step 6:** Recheck the injured part for feeling, warmth and color every few minutes.

# Apply an Anatomic Splint

**Step 1:** Check the scene and the victim.

**Step 2:** Support the injured area above and below the site of the injury.

**Step 3:** Check for feeling, warmth and color.

**Step 4:** Place several folded triangular bandages above and below the injured area.

**Step 5:** Tie triangular bandages securely.

**Step 6:** Recheck the injured part for feeling, warmth and color every few minutes.

# Apply a Sling

**Step 1:** Check the scene and the victim.

**Step 2:** Support the injured area above and below the site of the injury.

Leave the arm in the position you find it.

**Step 3:** Check for feeling, warmth and color.

**Step 4:** Place a triangular bandage under the injured arm and over the uninjured shoulder to form a sling.

## Step 5: Tie the ends of the sling at side of the neck.

Place pads of gauze under the knots to make it more comfortable for the victim.

## Step 6: Bind the injured area to the chest with a folded triangular bandage.

## Step 7: Recheck the injured part for feeling, warmth and color every few minutes.

# Apply a Rigid Splint

**Step 1:** Check the scene and the victim.

**Step 2:** Support the injured area above and below the site of the injury.

**Step 3:** Check for feeling, warmth and color.

**Step 4:** Place the rigid splint under the injured area and the joints that are above and below the injured area.

## Step 5: Tie several folded triangular bandages above and below the injured area.

## Step 6: Recheck the injured part for feeling, warmth and color every few minutes.

Immobilize above and below the site of the injury.

## SPECIAL SITUATIONS

Although head, neck and back injuries are only a small fraction of all injuries, they cause more than half the deaths. Each year, more than 2 million Americans suffer a head, neck or back injury. Most of them are males between the ages of 15 and 30. Motor vehicle accidents cause about half of all head, neck and back injuries. Falls, sports accidents and acts of violence are other causes.[64]

Injuries to the head, neck and back can cause paralysis, speech or memory problems or other disabling conditions. Injuries to the head, neck and back can damage bone and soft tissue, including the brain and spinal cord. Since generally only X-rays, CAT scans or MRIs can show the severity of a head, neck or back injury, you should always care for such an injury as if it were serious.

An injury to the brain can cause bleeding inside the skull. The blood can build up and cause pressure that can cause more damage. The first and most important signal of brain injury is a change in the level of the victim's consciousness. He or she may be dizzy or confused or may become unconscious.

The spine is a strong, flexible column of small bones that support the head and trunk. The spinal cord runs through the circular openings of the small bones, the vertebrae. The vertebrae are separated from each other by cushions of cartilage called disks. Nerves originating in the brain form branches extending to various parts of the body through openings in the vertebrae. Injuries to the back can fracture vertebrae and tear ligaments.

**Injuries to the head can rupture blood vessels in the brain. Pressure builds within the skull as blood accumulates, causing brain injury.**

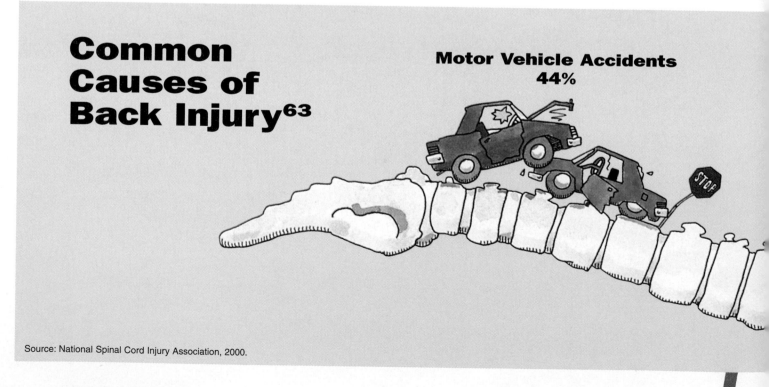

# Common Causes of Back Injury[63]

**Motor Vehicle Accidents 44%**

Source: National Spinal Cord Injury Association, 2000.

# WHEN TO SUSPECT HEAD, NECK AND BACK INJURIES

A fall from a height greater than that of the victim or any fall by an elderly person.

Any diving mishap.

A person found unconscious for unknown reasons.

Any motor vehicle accident involving a driver or passengers where severe blunt force to the head or chest, abdomen or pelvic area is possible.

Any injury that penetrates the head or chest, abdomen or pelvic area, such as a gunshot wound.

Any person thrown from a motor vehicle.

Any injury in which a victim's helmet is broken, including a motorcycle, bicycle, football or industrial helmet.

An incident involving a lightning strike or other incident where the victim is thrown.

**Falls 22%**

**Acts of Violence 24%**

**Sports Injuries 8% (two thirds from diving)**

**Other 2%**

7
Cervical

12
Thoracic

5
Lumbar

9
Sacrum
and Coccyx

C1
C2
C3
C4
C5
C6
C7
T1
T2
T3
T4
T5
T6
T7
T10
T11
T12
L1
L2
L3
L4
L5
S1
S2
S3
S4
S5

Sacrum
5 fused vertebrae

Coccyx
4 fused vertebrae

Injuries to the spine can paralyze or kill. The spine is a strong flexible column of small bones (vertebrae) that supports the head and trunk. The spinal cord runs through the center of these bones. Nerves originating in the brain form branches extending to various parts of the body through small openings in the vertebrae.

Nerve branches

Spinal cord

Intervertebral disk

Vertebrae

In some cases the vertebrae can shift and cut or squeeze the spinal cord. This can paralyze and even kill the victim.

When you are dealing with an injured person, think whether the forces involved in the injury were great enough to cause a head, neck or back injury. A victim may have fallen from a height or may have struck his or her head diving. The victim might have been in a motor vehicle accident and might not have been wearing a safety belt or might have been thrown from the vehicle. The victim might have been struck by lightning. The victim's back might have been pierced by a bullet that struck the spine. Always suspect a head, neck or back injury in a victim whose safety helmet has been broken by the injury or who is unconscious.

Besides the cause of the injury, certain signals suggest head, neck or back injury. They include a change in consciousness, problems with breathing and vision, inability to move a body part,

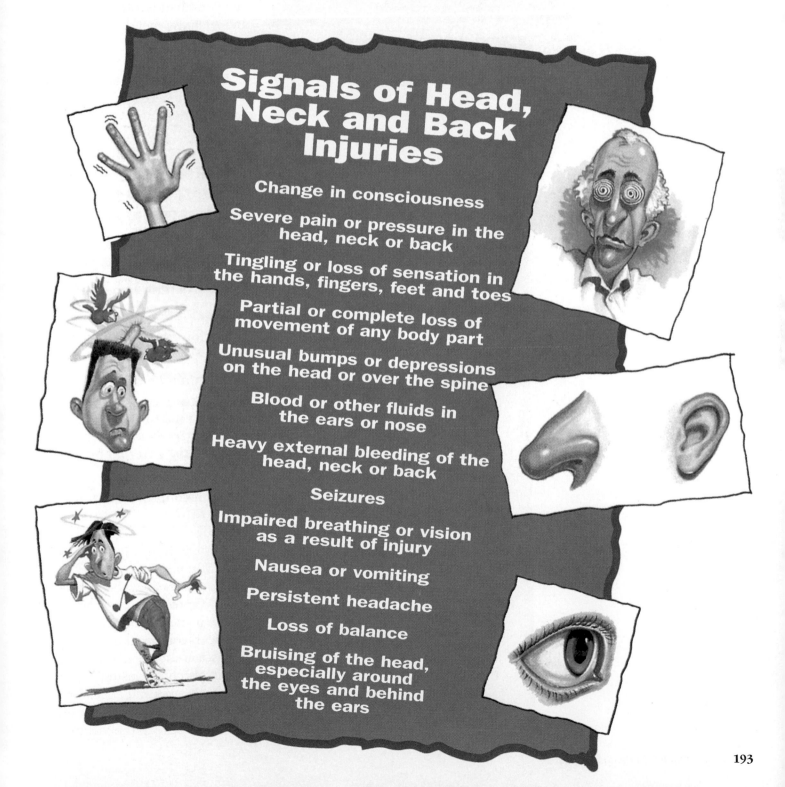

# Signals of Head, Neck and Back Injuries

**Change in consciousness**

**Severe pain or pressure in the head, neck or back**

**Tingling or loss of sensation in the hands, fingers, feet and toes**

**Partial or complete loss of movement of any body part**

**Unusual bumps or depressions on the head or over the spine**

**Blood or other fluids in the ears or nose**

**Heavy external bleeding of the head, neck or back**

**Seizures**

**Impaired breathing or vision as a result of injury**

**Nausea or vomiting**

**Persistent headache**

**Loss of balance**

**Bruising of the head, especially around the eyes and behind the ears**

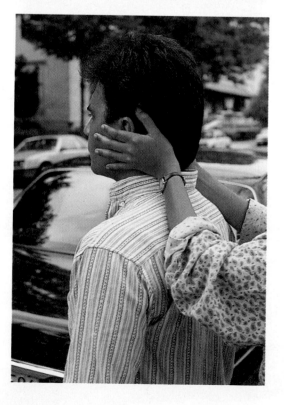

ongoing headache, nausea and vomiting, and loss of balance.

If you think a person has a head, neck or back injury, call 9-1-1 or the local emergency number. While you are waiting for EMS personnel to arrive, the best care you can give is to minimize movement of the victim's head and spine. Do this by placing your hands on both sides of the victim's head. Position the head gently in line with the body and support it in that position until EMS personnel arrive. If you feel resistance as you try to do this or it hurts the victim, stop. If the head is sharply turned to one side, do not try to move it. Support the head as you found it.

## GENERAL CARE FOR HEAD, NECK AND BACK INJURIES

**Minimize movement of the head, neck and back.**

**Maintain an open airway.**

**Check consciousness and breathing.**

**Control any external bleeding.**

**Keep the victim from getting chilled or overheated.**

The victim may become confused, drowsy or unconscious. Breathing may stop. The victim may be bleeding. If the victim is unconscious, you need to keep the airway open using the jaw-thrust maneuver and check breathing. You should control any severe bleeding and keep the victim from getting chilled or overheated. Remember, if you think the victim may have a head, neck or back injury, call 9-1-1 or the local emergency number.

Injuries to the chest may also result from falls, sports mishaps and crushing or penetrating forces. Chest injuries range from a simple broken rib to serious life-threatening injuries. Although painful, a simple broken rib is rarely life threatening. A victim with a broken rib will take small, shallow breaths because normal or deep breathing is painful. The victim will experience discomfort or pain at the site of the injury. The victim will usually try to ease the pain by supporting the area with a hand or arm. If the injury is serious, the victim will have trouble breathing. The victim's skin may appear flushed, pale or ashen and he or she may cough up blood. Always consider that a person with a serious chest injury may also have a back injury.

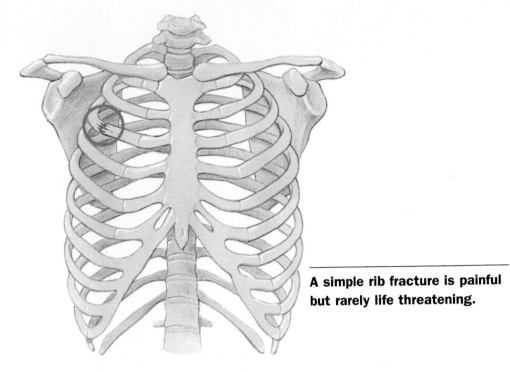

**A simple rib fracture is painful but rarely life threatening.**

If you suspect injured ribs, have the victim rest in a position that will make breathing easier. Binding the victim's arm to the chest on the injured side will help support the injured area and make breathing more comfortable. You can use an object, such as a pillow or folded blanket, to support and immobilize the area. If you think the injury is serious or the spine has also been injured, have the victim lie flat. Continue to watch the victim until EMS personnel arrive and take over.

The large, heavy bones of the hip are called the pelvis. Like the chest, injury to the pelvic bones can range from simple to life threatening. Because these large bones help to protect important organs inside the body, severe forces can cause heavy internal bleeding. Although a serious injury may be immediately obvious, some may develop over time.

Because an injury to the pelvis can also injure the lower spine, it is best not to move the victim. If possible, try to keep the victim lying flat. Watch for signals of internal bleeding and take steps to minimize shock until EMS personnel arrive.

**When a rib fracture occurs, use a pillow or folded blanket to support and immobilize the injured area.**

# SUDDEN ILLNESS

It is usually obvious when someone is injured and needs care. The victim may be able to tell you what happened and what hurts. Checking the victim also gives you clues about what might be wrong. When someone becomes suddenly ill, however, it is not as easy to tell what is wrong. At times there are no warning signals to give clues about what is happening. At other times, the signals only confirm that something is wrong. In either case the signals of a sudden illness are often confusing. You may find it difficult to determine if the victim's condition is an emergency and whether to call 9-1-1 or the local emergency number.

## RECOGNIZING SUDDEN ILLNESS

Although there are many different types of sudden illnesses, they often have similar signals. Victims generally look ill. The signals can include a change in consciousness, such as feeling lightheaded, dizzy or becoming unconscious and nausea or vomiting. The victim may have difficulty speaking or complain of numbness or paralysis. You may also see changes in breathing. The victim may have trouble breathing or may not be breathing normally. The victim's skin may become pale, ashen or flushed and the victim may be sweating. The victim may be in pain or have difficulty moving.

Besides the physical signals you see, you may also be able to get some clues by looking at the victim's location and at what he or she was doing when the illness started. For example, if someone

### SIGNALS OF SUDDEN ILLNESS

**When a person becomes suddenly ill, he or she often looks and feels sick. Common signals include—**

• **Feeling lightheaded, dizzy, confused or weak.**

• **Changes in skin color (pale, ashen or flushed skin) or sweating.**

• **Nausea or vomiting.**

• **Diarrhea.**

**Some sudden illnesses may also include—**

• **Changes in consciousness.**

• **Seizures.**

• **Paralysis or inability to move.**

• **Slurred speech.**

• **Difficulty seeing.**

• **Severe headache.**

• **Trouble breathing.**

• **Persistent pressure or pain.**

working in a hot environment suddenly becomes ill, it would make sense to suspect the illness is the result of the heat. If someone suddenly feels ill or behaves strangely and is attempting to take medication, the medication may be a clue to what is wrong.

## IF A PERSON BECOMES SUDDENLY ILL, DON'T SECOND-GUESS, CALL EMS.

For example, the person may take medication for a heart condition, epilepsy or diabetes.

With some sudden illnesses, you might not be sure whether to call 9-1-1 or the local emergency number for help. Sometimes the signals come and go. However, if you cannot sort the problem out quickly and easily or if you have any doubts about the severity of the illness, call 9-1-1 or your local emergency number for help. It is better to be safe than sorry.

## GENERAL CARE FOR SUDDEN ILLNESS

Usually you will not know the exact cause of the sudden illness, but this should not keep you from providing appropriate care. This is because you will initially care for the signals present, not for any specific condition. In the few cases where you may know that the person has a medical condi-

# SEIZURES

When the normal workings of the brain are disrupted by injury, disease, fever or infection, the electrical activity of the brain becomes irregular. This can cause a loss of body control known as a seizure. Seizures may be caused by extreme heat, a diabetic condition or an injury to the brain.

Seizures may be caused by an acute or chronic condition. The chronic condition is known as epilepsy. Over 2 million Americans have epilepsy.[65] Epilepsy is usually controlled with medication. Still, some people with epilepsy have seizures from time to time. Others who go a long time without a seizure may think the condition has gone away and stop taking their medication. These people may then have a seizure again.

The person may experience an aura before the seizure occurs. An aura is an unusual sensation or feeling such as a visual hallucination; strange sound, taste or smell; or an urgent need to get to safety. If the person recognizes the aura, he or she may have time to tell bystanders and sit down before the seizure occurs.

Seizures range from a blank stare or period of distorted sensation where the victim is unable to respond, so that others may mistake the seizure for daydreaming, to sudden, uncontrolled muscular contractions (convulsion) lasting several minutes. Infants and young children are at risk for seizures brought on by high fever. These are called febrile (heat-induced) seizures.

Although it may be frightening to see someone unexpectedly having a seizure, you should remember that most seizures last only for a few minutes and the person usually recovers without problems. While most seizures are not life threatening, call 9-1-1 or the local emergency number if the seizure lasts more than 5 minutes; the seizure recurs; the victim is pregnant; the victim is diabetic; or the victim becomes injured or shows other life-threatening conditions. Care for the person until help arrives by protecting the victim from injury and keeping the airway open. Do not insert any item into the victim's mouth. If there is fluid, such as saliva, blood or vomit, in the victim's mouth, roll him or her on one side so that the fluid can drain from the mouth.

# DON'T SECOND GUESS— CALL EMS

## Call 9-1-1 or the local emergency number if the victim—

**Is unconscious, unusually confused or seems to be losing consciousness.**

**Has trouble breathing or is breathing in a strange way.**

**Has persistent chest discomfort or pressure.**

**Has pressure or discomfort in the abdomen that does not go away.**

**Is vomiting or passing blood.**

**Has a seizure lasting more than 5 minutes or has multiple seizures.**

**Has a seizure and is pregnant.**

**Has a seizure and is diabetic.**

**Has a severe headache or slurred speech.**

**Appears to have been poisoned.**

**Has injuries to the head, neck or back.**

tion, such as diabetes, epilepsy or a heart condition, the care you provide may be slightly different. This care may involve helping the person take medication for his or her specific illness.

The care for sudden illnesses follows the same general guidelines as for any emergency. First, check the scene for any clues about what might be wrong. Then check the victim. Make sure 9-1-1 or the local emergency number has been called for any life-threatening conditions. Care for any life-threatening conditions such as: unconsciousness, trouble breathing, no breathing, no signs of circulation, severe bleeding or severe chest pain. If the victim vomits, position the victim on his or her side.

When providing care, always care for life-threatening conditions before those that are not life threatening. Help the victim rest comfortably. Keep the victim from getting chilled or overheated. Reassure the victim because he or she may be anxious or frightened. Watch for changes in consciousness and breathing. If the victim is conscious, ask if he or she has any medical conditions or is taking any medication.

## SPECIAL CONDITIONS

When someone suddenly loses consciousness and then re-awakens, he or she may simply have fainted. Fainting itself is not usually harmful and the victim will usually quickly recover. Lower the victim to the ground or other flat surface and position him or her on the back. If possible, elevate the victim's legs 8 to 12 inches. Loosen any tight clothing, such as a tie or collar. Check to make sure the victim is breathing. Do not give the victim anything to eat or drink. If the victim vomits, reposition to his or her side.

Since you will not be able to tell whether the fainting is a signal of a more serious condition, you should call 9-1-1 or the local emergency number.

Some illnesses that seem to come on suddenly are really caused by long-term conditions. These causes include degenerative diseases, such as heart and lung diseases. There may be a

If a victim of a diabetic emergency is conscious, give him or her fluids containing sugar.

# CARE FOR SUDDEN ILLNESS

## Care for any life-threatening conditions first. Then—

- Help the victim rest comfortably.

- Keep the victim from getting chilled or overheated.

- Reassure the victim.

- Watch for changes in consciousness and breathing.

- Do not give anything to eat or drink unless the victim is fully conscious.

## If the victim—

**Vomits**—Place him or her on the side so that you can clear the mouth.

**Faints**—Position him or her on the back and elevate the legs 8 to 10 inches if you do not suspect a head, neck or back injury.

**Has a diabetic emergency**—Give the conscious victim some type of sugar, preferably in liquid form, such as orange or apple juice, non-diet soda or 2–3 teaspoons of sugar dissolved in a glass of water.

**Has a seizure**—Do not hold or restrain the person or place anything between the victim's teeth. Remove any nearby objects that might cause injury. Cushion the victim's head using folded clothing or a small pillow.

**Has a severe allergic reaction**—Assist the victim with his or her medication, which may be available as a single-dose epinephrine "pen."

# Diabetes: A Silent Killer

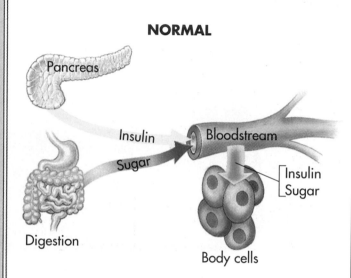

**NORMAL**

Pancreas

Insulin

Bloodstream

Sugar

Insulin
Sugar

Digestion

Body cells

**DIABETIC**

Pancreas

Insulin

Sugar
Bloodstream

Sugar

Digestion

Body cells

Diabetes is a leading cause of death in the United States, affecting hundreds of thousands of people. Diabetes can lead to other medical conditions such as blindness, nerve disease, kidney disease, heart disease and stroke. According to the American Diabetes Association, diabetes is the inability of the body to convert sugar from food into energy.[66]

When you do daily activities like exercising, the cells in your body need sugar as a source of energy. The cells receive this energy during digestion, when the body breaks food into sugars. The sugar then becomes absorbed into the blood with the help of a hormone called insulin. Insulin is produced in the body and takes sugar into the cells. For the body to function properly, there has to be a balance of insulin and sugar in the body or the cells will starve.

Almost 16 million people in the United States have diabetes; among this group, more than 5 million people are unaware that they have the disease.[67] When insulin is not produced or used in the proper amount, diabetes occurs. There are two major types of diabetes: Type I,

insulin-dependent diabetes and Type II, noninsulin-dependent diabetes. Diabetes is a chronic disease that currently has no cure.

Type I diabetes affects about 1 million Americans. This type of diabetes usually begins in childhood and is often called juvenile diabetes. This type of diabetes occurs when the body produces little or no insulin. Therefore most insulin-dependent diabetics have to inject insulin into their bodies daily.

The exact cause of juvenile diabetes is not known. Warning signals of Type I diabetes include the following:[68]

- Frequent urination
- Increased hunger and thirst
- Unexpected weight loss
- Irritability
- Weakness and fatigue

The most common type of diabetes is Type II diabetes, which affects about 90-95 percent of individuals with diabetes. This condition is called adult-onset diabetes and usually occurs in adults, but also can occur in children who are likely to be overweight. With Type II, noninsulin-dependent diabetes, the body makes insulin but not in the neces-

# DIABETIC EMERGENCIES

## DIABETIC COMA (HYPERGLYCEMIA)

## INSULIN REACTION (HYPOGLYCEMIA)

sary amounts or the body becomes resistant to the insulin produced.

According to the American Diabetes Association,[69] "Medical experts do not know the exact cause of Type II diabetes. They do know Type II diabetes runs in families. A person can inherit a tendency to get Type II diabetes, but it usually takes another factor, such as obesity, to bring on the disease."

Individuals from certain racial and ethnic backgrounds are known to be at greater risk for diabetes. For example, Type II diabetes is more common among African Americans, Latinos, Asians, certain Native Americans and Pacific Islanders.

Warning signals of Type II diabetes include the following:[70]
- Any signals of Type I diabetes
- Frequent infections, especially involving the skin, gums and bladder
- Blurred vision
- Numbness in legs, feet and fingers
- Cuts/bruises that are slow to heal
- Itching

Often people with Type II diabetes have no signals.

It is important for all individuals with diabetes to monitor their exercise and diet. Self-monitoring for blood sugar levels is a valuable tool. Insulin-dependent diabetics must monitor their use of in-

sulin. If a diabetic does not control these factors, an imbalance between insulin and sugar in the body can create a diabetic emergency. Signals and symptoms of a diabetic emergency include the following:
- Changes in the level of consciousness
- Rapid breathing and pulse
- Feeling and looking ill

For more information about diabetes, contact the American Diabetes Association at 1-800-DIABETES or at customerservice@diabetes.org

For information specifically about Type I diabetes, contact the Juvenile Diabetes Foundation at 1-800-JDF-CURE or at info@jdf.org hormone imbalance, such as in diabetes. The victim could have epilepsy, a condition that causes seizures. An allergy can cause a sudden and sometimes dangerous reaction to certain substances. When checking a victim, look for a medical bracelet, necklace or anklet indicating the victim has a chronic condition.

People who are diabetic sometimes become ill because there is too much or too little sugar in their blood. The signals of a diabetic emergency are the same as for any other sudden illness. They require the same care. You may know the victim is a diabetic or the victim may tell you he or she is a diabetic. Often diabetics know what is wrong and will ask for something with sugar in it. They may carry some form of sugar with them in case they need it.

If the victim is conscious and can take food or fluids, give him or her sugar, preferably in liquid form. If the victim is conscious and unable to swallow, do not put anything, liquid or solid, into the victim's mouth.[71] Instead, immediately call 9-1-1 or the local emergency number. Most fruit juices and non-diet soft drinks have enough sugar to be effective. You can also give table sugar dissolved in a glass of water. If the person's problem is low blood sugar, sugar will help quickly. If the problem is too much sugar, the sugar will not

# FAINTING

**O**ne common signal of sudden illness is losing consciousness, such as when a person faints. Fainting is a temporary loss of consciousness. A person who is about to faint often becomes pale, begins to sweat and then loses consciousness and collapses.

Fainting occurs when there is an insufficient supply of blood to the brain for a short period of time. This condition results from a widening of the blood vessels in the body, which causes blood to drain away from the brain. A person who feels weak or dizzy may prevent a fainting spell by lying down or sitting with the head level with the knees.

Usually the victim of fainting recovers quickly with no lasting effects. But what appears to be a simple case of fainting may actually be a signal of a more serious condition. The victim may also be injured from falling. You should always call 9-1-1 or the local emergency number. If it happens to you, even just once, be sure to tell your health-care provider.

**To care for a person who has fainted, place him or her on the back, elevate the feet and loosen any restrictive clothing, such as a belt, tie or collar.**

cause any further harm. If the person does not feel better within about 5 minutes after taking sugar, call 9-1-1 or your local emergency number. If you cannot find sugar immediately, do not spend time looking for it; call 9-1-1 or the local emergency number.

If the person is unconscious or about to lose consciousness, do not give him or her anything by mouth. Instead, call 9-1-1 or the local emergency number and care for the victim in the same way as you would care for any unconscious person. This includes making sure the person's airway is clear of vomit and checking breathing and signs of circulation until help arrives.

Stroke is another cause of sudden illness that requires prompt medical care. A person who has had a stroke will show many of the common signals of other sudden illnesses.

Care for the victim as you would for anyone else who is suddenly ill. Help the victim rest comfortably. Comfort the victim. He or she might not understand what has happened. Do not give anything to eat or drink. If the victim is unconscious or drooling or is having difficulty swallowing, place him or her on one side to help drain fluids from the mouth. Have someone call 9-1-1 or the local emergency number while you take care of the victim.

Sometimes a person who becomes suddenly ill may have a seizure. Although it may be frightening to see someone unexpectedly having a seizure, you can easily help care for the person. Remember that he or she cannot control the seizure. Do not try to stop the seizure. Do not hold or restrain the person.

**IF A PERSON BECOMES SUDDENLY ILL, CARE FOR ANY LIFE-THREATENING CONDITIONS FIRST.**

Care for the seizure victim as you would for any unconscious person. To protect the seizure victim from injury, remove any nearby objects that might cause injury. Protect the victim's head by placing a thin cushion under it. Folded clothing makes an adequate cushion. If there is fluid in the victim's mouth, such as saliva, blood or vomit, roll him or her on one side so that the fluid drains from the mouth.

Do not try to place anything between the victim's teeth. People having seizures rarely bite their tongues or cheeks with enough force to cause any significant bleeding. However, some blood may be present.

When the seizure is over, the victim usually begins to breathe normally. He or she may be drowsy and disoriented. Check to see if the victim was injured during the seizure. Be reassuring and comforting. If the seizure occurred in public, the victim may be embarrassed and self-conscious. Ask bystanders not to crowd around the victim. He or she will be tired and want to rest. Stay with the victim until he or she is fully conscious and aware of the surroundings.

If the victim is known to have occasional seizures, you do not have to call EMS. The victim will usually recover from a seizure in a few minutes. However, call 9-1-1 or the local emergency number[72] if—

- The seizure lasts more than 5 minutes.
- The victim has multiple seizures.
- The victim appears to be injured.
- The victim is pregnant.
- The victim is a diabetic.

Having to deal with a sudden illness can be scary, especially when you do not know what is wrong. Do not hesitate to provide care. Remember, you do not have to know the cause to help. As you can see, the signals for sudden illnesses are very similar to other conditions and the care involves skills that you already know.

NING

ICKY

CREEPY

CRAWLY

ITCHY

A poison is a substance that causes injury or illness if it gets into the body. Some poisons can cause death. There are four ways a person can be poisoned: by swallowing the poison, by breathing it, by absorbing it through the skin and by having it injected into the body.

Approximately 900,000 visits due to poisoning are made to hospital emergency departments each year in the United States. In 1998, more than 92 percent of all poisonings took place in the home and 53 percent involved children under the age of 6 years.[73] Poisoning deaths in children under age 5 have dropped in the last 30 years, but poisoning deaths among adults 18 and older have greatly increased.

The decrease in child poisonings is the result of packaging for drugs and medications that makes these substances harder for children to get into. It is also a result of preventive actions by parents and others who care for children.

The increase in adult poisoning deaths is linked to an increase in suicides and increases in drug-related poisonings.

Poisons a person can swallow include foods, such as certain mushrooms and shellfish; alcohol; medications, such as aspirin; household and garden items, such as cleaning products and pesticides; and certain plants. Many substances not poisonous in small amounts are poisonous in larger amounts. Misusing and abusing certain drugs, such as sleeping

# Watch Your Step

**Annually, millions of people suffer from contact with poisonous plants.**

How many times have you been told, "Watch your step...there's poison ivy?" Would you know what to look for? Could you identify it before you started itching? Millions of people each year suffer from contact with poisonous plants such as poison ivy, poison oak and poison sumac.

Most ill effects of contact with poisonous plants can be avoided by removing exposed clothing and washing the exposed area thoroughly with soap and water as soon as possible after contact. If a rash or weeping sore has already begun to develop,

**Poison Ivy**

John Shaw/Tom Stack & Associates

**Poison Sumac**

John Shaw/Tom Stack & Associates

put a paste of baking soda and water on the area several times a day to reduce the discomfort. Calamine lotion and antihistamines, such as Benadryl™, may also help dry up the sores. If the condition gets worse and affects large areas of the body or the face, see a health-care provider. It may be necessary to give anti-inflammatory drugs, such as cor-

ticosteroids or other medications, to relieve discomfort. Be sure to wash clothing exposed to plant oils since the oils can linger on fabric. Wash your hands thoroughly after handling exposed clothing. Also wash your hands after touching exposed pets.

**Poison Oak**

Walt Anderson/Tom Stack & Associates

pills, tranquilizers and alcohol, can also result in poisoning. Combinations of certain substances, such as drugs and alcohol, can be poisonous, although if taken by themselves they might not cause harm.

Poisoning can also result from breathing toxic fumes. Inhaled poisons may be gases, such as carbon monoxide from an engine or car exhaust; carbon dioxide from wells and sewers; and chlorine, found in many swimming pools. Inhaled poisons also include fumes from household products, such as glues, paints and cleaners and fumes from drugs, such as crack cocaine.

An absorbed poison enters the body through the skin. Absorbed poisons come from plants, such as poison ivy, poison oak and poison sumac, as well as from fertilizers and pesticides used in lawn and plant care. Injected poisons enter the body through bites or stings of insects, spiders, ticks, some marine life, snakes and other animals or through drugs or medications injected with a hypodermic needle.

How will you know if someone who is ill has been poisoned? Look for clues about what has happened. Try to get information from the victim or from any bystanders. If you suspect that the victim's condition is caused by some form of poisoning, call your Poison Control Center, 9-1-1 or the local emergency number. Follow their direction. If the victim becomes violent or threatening, retreat to safety and wait for help to arrive.

As you check the scene, be aware of any unusual odors, flames, smoke, open or spilled containers, an open medicine cabinet, an overturned or damaged plant or other signals of possible poisoning. The signals of poisoning include nausea, vomiting, diarrhea, chest or abdominal pain, trouble breathing, sweating, changes in consciousness and seizures. Other signals of poisoning are burns around the lips, tongue or on the skin. You may also suspect a poisoning based on any information you have from or about the victim.

If you suspect someone has swallowed a poison, try to find out—

• What type of poison it was.
• How much was taken.
• When it was taken.
• How much the victim weighs.

This information can help you and others provide the most appropriate care.

Follow these general guidelines if you suspect someone has been poisoned:

• Check the scene to make sure it is safe to approach and to gather clues about what happened.
• Remove the victim from the source of poison, if necessary.
• Check the victim's level of consciousness, breathing and signs of circulation.
• Care for any life-threatening conditions.
• If the victim is conscious, ask questions to get more information.
• Look for any containers and take them with you to the telephone.
• Call the Poison Control Center, 9-1-1 or the local emergency number.
• Follow the directions of the Poison Control Center or the EMS dispatcher.

Do not give the victim anything to eat or drink unless medical professionals tell you to. If you do not know what the poison was and the victim vomits, save some

# MORE THAN 92 PERCENT OF ALL POISONINGS TAKE PLACE IN THE HOME.

**Ingestion**

**Inhalation**

**Absorption**

**Injection**

**A poison can enter the body in four ways: ingestion, inhalation, absorption and injection.**

# Poison Control Centers

Poison Control Centers (PCCs) help people deal with poisons. There are PCCs all over the United States. Many centers are in the emergency departments of large hospitals. The people who staff these centers have access to information about almost all poisonous substances. They will tell you how to counteract the poison. Keep your local PCC telephone number posted by your telephone. The number will be in your telephone directory. You can also get it from your doctor, a local hospital or your local EMS system.

In 1998, PCCs answered over 2.2 million calls about poisonings.[74] Many poisonings can be cared for without the help of EMS personnel, so PCCs help reduce the workload of the EMS system. If the victim is conscious, call your local or regional PCC first. The center staff will tell you what care to give and whether to call for an ambulance.

If the victim is unconscious or if you do not know your PCC number, call 9-1-1 or the local emergency number. The dispatcher may be able to link you with the PCC. The dispatcher may also listen in on your talk with the PCC and send an ambulance if needed.

When someone has swallowed a poison, the PCC may tell you to make the victim vomit by giving syrup of ipecac (about 2 tablespoons). You can buy syrup of ipecac at your local drug store. It usually comes in a 30-milliliter bottle. Two tablespoons, followed by two glasses of water, is the normal dose for a person over 12 years of age. For children aged 1 to 12, the normal dose is 1 tablespoon followed by two glasses of water. The victim usually vomits within 20 minutes. Young children often will not take syrup of ipecac, so it may have to be given in the hospital. **Never use syrup of ipecac before calling the Poison Control Center.**

There are some instances when you should not induce vomiting.[75] This is why you should call the PCC for advice. Do not make the victim vomit if he or she has swallowed a corrosive substance (an acid or alkali) or a petroleum product such as kerosene or gasoline. Corrosive substances burn tissues and, if vomited, can burn the esophagus, throat and mouth.

Since vomiting removes only about half the poison, the PCC may advise you to counteract the remaining poison with activated charcoal. You can buy it in both liquid and powdered forms from drug stores. Before use, the powder should be mixed in water to form a solution with the consistency of a milk shake. For a person over 12 years of age, follow the directions on the bottle. Young children usually will not take activated charcoal, so it is given to them in the hospital. **Never use activated charcoal before calling the Poison Control Center.**

---

**Syrup of ipecac is used to induce vomiting in victims who have swallowed certain kinds of poisons. Activated charcoal is used to absorb swallowed poisons.**

# IF YOU THINK SOMEONE HAS BEEN POISONED, CALL YOUR POISON CONTROL CENTER OR LOCAL EMERGENCY NUMBER AND FOLLOW THEIR DIRECTIONS.

of the vomit. The hospital may analyze it to identify the poison.

Just as it may be difficult to know if someone has swallowed poison, it may be difficult to tell if someone who is ill has been breathing toxic fumes. Toxic fumes come from a variety of sources. They may have an odor or be odor-free. A commonly inhaled poison is carbon monoxide. It is produced by gasoline-burning engines, defective cooking equipment, fires and charcoal grills.

When someone breathes in toxic fumes, the victim's skin may turn pale or ashen. This may mean a lack of oxygen. If it is safe for you to do so, get the victim of inhaled poison to fresh air. All victims of inhaled poison need fresh air as soon as possible.

If poisons, such as wet chemicals, get on the skin, flush the affected area with large amounts of water. Have someone else call 9-1-1 or the local emergency number. Keep flushing the area until EMS personnel arrive.

Dry chemicals, such as lime, should be brushed off with gloved hands. Take care not to get any in your eyes or the eyes of the victim or any bystanders.

To care for skin that has come in contact with a poison, immediately flush the affected area with water.

If someone is stung by an insect, remove the stinger. Scrape it away from the skin with your fingernail or a plastic card, such as a credit card.

**Black Widow**

Rob Planck/Tom Stack & Associates

## BITES AND STINGS

Insect stings are painful, but they are rarely fatal. Some people, however, have a severe allergic reaction to an insect sting. This allergic reaction may result in a breathing emergency.

**Bites from the black widow spider and the brown recluse spider can make you sick or be fatal. Because both spiders prefer dark, out-of-the-way places, the victim may not know that he or she has been bitten until he or she starts to feel ill or notices a bite mark or swelling.**

**Brown Recluse**

Ann Moreton/Tom Stack & Associates

Rob Planck/Tom Stack & Associates

**Scorpion**

If someone is stung by an insect, remove the stinger. Scrape it away from the skin with your fingernail or a plastic card, such as a credit or bank card, or use tweezers. If you use tweezers, grasp the stinger, not the venom sac. Wash the site with soap and water. Cover it to keep it clean. Apply a cold pack to the area to reduce the pain and swelling. Watch the victim for signals of an allergic reaction.

Scorpions live in dry regions of the southwestern United States. They live under rocks, logs and the bark of certain trees and are most active at night. Only a few species of scorpions have a sting that can cause death.

There are also only two spiders in the United States whose bite can make you seriously sick or be fatal. These are the black widow spider and the brown recluse spider. The black widow spider is black with a reddish hourglass shape on the underside of its body. The brown recluse spider is light brown with a darker brown, violin-shaped marking on the top of its body. Both spiders prefer dark, out-of-the-way places. Bites usually occur on the hands and arms of people reaching into places such as wood, rock and brush piles or rummaging in dark garages and attics. Often, the vic-

**The bites of only a few species of scorpions found in the United States can be fatal.**

# Lyme Disease

Nymph

Adult

Lyme disease is an illness that people get from the bite of an infected tick. Lyme disease is affecting a growing number of people in the United States. Although Lyme disease has been reported in almost every state, 90 percent of cases of Lyme disease in the past decade have been reported in ten states: New York, Connecticut, Pennsylvania, New Jersey, Wisconsin, Rhode Island, Maryland, Massachusetts, Minnesota and Delaware.[76] Because Lyme disease appears to be spreading, everyone should take precautions to protect against it.

Not all ticks carry Lyme disease. Lyme disease is spread mainly by a type of tick that commonly attaches itself to field mice and deer. It is sometimes called a deer tick. The tick is found around branches and in wooded and grassy areas. Like all ticks, it attaches itself to any warm-blooded animal that brushes by it, including humans. A deer tick can attach to you without your knowledge. Many people who develop Lyme disease cannot recall having been bitten.

Deer ticks are very tiny and difficult to see. They are much smaller than the common dog tick or wood tick. They can be as small as a poppy seed or the head of a pin. Adult deer ticks are only as large as a grape seed. Because of the tiny size of the tick, a tick bite is usually painless.

You can get Lyme disease from the bite of an infected tick at any time of the year. However, in northern states, the risk is greatest between May and late August, when ticks are most active and people spend more time outdoors. Recent studies indicate that the tick must remain embedded in human skin for about 48 hours to transmit Lyme disease.[77] Always check for ticks immediately after outdoor activities. All clothing should be washed. Be sure to check pets because they can develop signals of Lyme disease as well as carry ticks into the house, where they can then attach themselves to unsuspecting people.

The first signal of infection may appear a few days or a few weeks after a tick bite. Typically, a rash starts as a small red area at the site of the bite. It may spread up to 7 inches across. In fair-skinned people, the center is lighter in color and the outer edges are red and raised. This sometimes gives the rash a bull's-eye appearance. In dark-skinned people, the area may look black and blue, like a bruise.

Other signals of Lyme disease include fever, headache, weakness and joint and muscle pain similar to the signals of flu. These signals might develop slowly and might not occur at the same time as the rash. In fact, you can have Lyme disease without developing a rash.

Lyme disease can get worse if not treated. In its advanced stages, it may cause arthritis, numbness, memory loss, problems in seeing or hearing, high fever and stiff neck. Some of these signals could indicate problems with the brain or nervous system. An irregular or rapid heartbeat could indicate heart problems.

If you find a tick, remove it by pulling steadily and firmly. Grasp the tick with fine-tipped tweezers, as close to the skin as possible, and pull slowly. If you do not have tweezers, use a glove, plastic wrap or a piece of paper to protect your fingers. If you use your bare fingers, wash your hands immediately. Do not try to burn a tick off with a hot match or burning cigarette. Do not use other home remedies, like coating the tick with Vaseline or nail polish or pricking it with a pin.

Once the tick is removed, wash the area immediately with soap and water. If an antiseptic or antibiotic ointment is available, apply it to prevent wound infection. Observe the site periodically thereafter.

If you cannot remove the tick or if parts of the tick stay in your skin, obtain medical care. If a rash or flu-like symptoms develop, seek medical help. A physician will usually use antibiotics to treat Lyme disease. Antibiotics work best and most quickly when taken early. If you suspect Lyme disease, do not delay seeking treatment. Treatment is slower and less effective in advanced stages.

More information on Lyme disease may be available from your local or state health department. Be sure to ask about current recommendations for the Lyme disease vaccine.

Michael Weisman, M.D./Fran Heyl Associates

**A person with Lyme disease may develop a rash.**

Bernard Funival/Fran Heyl Associates

**A deer tick can be as small as the head of a pin.**

tim will not know that he or she has been bitten until he or she starts to feel ill or notices a bite mark or swelling.

Signals of spider bites and scorpion stings also are similar to those of other sudden illnesses. However, if the person knows he or she has been bitten or stung, this might help identify the cause of the problem. The signals include nausea, vomiting, trouble breathing or swallowing, salivating much more than normal, sweating, severe pain in the sting or bite area and a mark indicating a possible bite or sting and swelling of the area.

If someone has been stung by a scorpion or bitten by a spider he or she thinks is a black widow or brown recluse, wash the wound, apply a cold pack to the site and get medical help immediately. Antivenin is available for black widow bites and for scorpion stings. Antivenin is medication that blocks the effects of the poisonous venom.

Snakebites kill very few people in the United States. Of the 7,000 people bitten annually in the United States, fewer than 15 die.[78] Most snakebites occur near the home, not in the wild. Rattlesnakes account for most snakebites and nearly all deaths from snakebites. Most deaths occur because the victim has an allergic reaction, is in poor health or because too much time passes before he or she receives medical care.

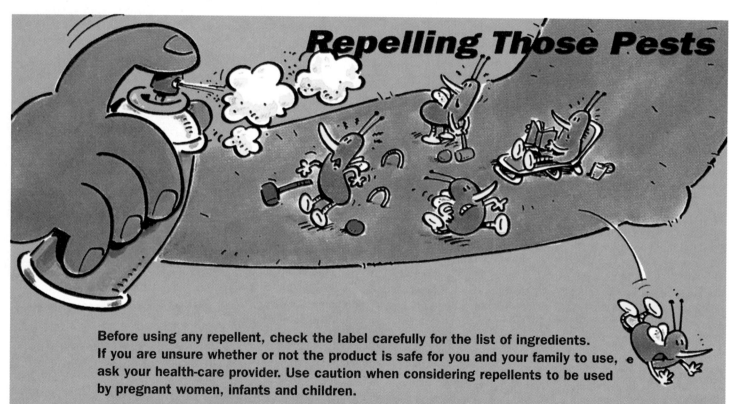

# Repelling Those Pests

**Before using any repellent, check the label carefully for the list of ingredients. If you are unsure whether or not the product is safe for you and your family to use, ask your health-care provider. Use caution when considering repellents to be used by pregnant women, infants and children.**

If you use a repellent, follow these general rules:

- Keep all repellents out of the reach of children.

- To apply repellent to the face, first spray it on your hands and then apply it from your hands to your face. Avoid sensitive areas, such as the lips and the eyes.

- Never use repellents on an open wound or irritated skin.

- Use repellents sparingly. One application will last 4 to 8 hours. Heavier or more frequent applications will not increase effectiveness.

- If you suspect you are having a reaction to a repellent, wash the treated skin immediately and call your health-care provider.

- Never put repellents on children's hands. They may put them in their eyes or mouth.

**For current information about pesticides, contact the National Pesticide Telecommunications Network (NPTN) at http://nptn.orst.org or at 1-800-858-7378 (6:30 a.m. to 4:30 p.m. Pacific Time, 7 days/week, except holidays).**

You hear all sorts of care recommended for snakebites. To care for someone bitten by a snake, wash the wound and immobilize the injured area, keeping it lower than the heart, if possible. Call 9-1-1 or the local emergency number. Do not apply ice to a snakebite. Do not cut the wound. Do not apply a tourniquet. Do not use electric shock, such as from a car battery. If necessary, carry a victim who must be taken to a medical facility or have him or her walk slowly.

If you know the victim cannot get emergency medical care within 30 minutes, consider suctioning the wound using a snakebite kit, if one is available. People at risk of snakebites in the wild (away from medical care) should carry a snakebite kit and know how to use its contents.

The bite of a domestic or wild animal can cause infection and soft tissue injury. The most seri-

**Portuguese Man-of-War**

**Sea Anemone**

**Jellyfish**

**The painful sting of some marine animals can cause serious problems.**

**Sting Ray**

# Caring for Bites and Stings

## INSECT BITES

### Signals

Stinger may be present

Pain

Swelling

Possible allergic reaction

### Care

Remove stinger— Scrape it away or use tweezers.

Wash wound.

Cover.

Apply a cold pack. Watch for signals of allergic reaction.

## SPIDER/SCORPION BITE STING

### Signals

Bite mark

Swelling

Pain

Nausea and vomiting

Trouble breathing or swallowing

### Care

Wash wound.

Apply a cold pack.

Get medical care to receive antivenin.

Call local emergency number, if necessary.

## MARINE LIFE STINGS

### Signals

Possible marks

Pain

Swelling

Possible allergic reaction

### Care

If jellyfish—soak area in vinegar.

If stingray—soak area in nonscalding hot water until pain goes away. Clean and bandage wound.

Call local emergency number, if necessary.

## SNAKE BITES

### Signals

Bite mark

Pain

### Care

Wash wound.

Keep bitten part still, and lower than the heart.

Call local emergency number.

## ANIMAL BITES

### Signals

Bite mark

Bleeding

### Care

If bleeding is minor, wash wound.

Control bleeding.

Apply antibiotic ointment.

Cover.

Get medical attention if wound bleeds severely or if you suspect animal has rabies.

Call local emergency number or contact animal control personnel.

# SNAKEBITES KILL VERY FEW PEOPLE IN THE UNITED STATES... MOST SNAKEBITES OCCUR NEAR THE HOME, NOT IN THE WILD.

ous possible result is rabies. Rabies is transmitted through the saliva of diseased animals, such as skunks, bats, raccoons, cats, dogs, cattle and foxes.

Animals with rabies may act strangely. For example, animals usually active at night, such as raccoons, may be active in the daytime. A wild animal that usually tries to avoid people might not run from you. Rabid animals may drool, appear partially paralyzed or act irritable, mean or strangely quiet. Do not pet or feed wild animals and do not touch the body of a dead animal.

If not treated, rabies is fatal. Anyone bitten by an animal that might have rabies must get medical attention. To prevent rabies, the victim receives a series of vaccine injections to build up immunity that will help fight the disease.

If someone is bitten by an animal, try to get him or her away from the animal without putting

**There are four kinds of poisonous snakes found in the United States.**

**Rattlesnake**

**Water Moccasin**

**Copperhead**

**Coral Snake**

yourself in danger. Do not try to stop, hold or catch the animal. If the wound is minor, wash it with soap and water. Then control any bleeding and apply an antibiotic ointment and a dressing. Get medical attention if you suspect the animal might have rabies. Watch for signals of infection.

If the wound is bleeding seriously, control the bleeding first. Do not clean the wound. Get medical attention. The wound will be properly cleaned at a medical facility.

If possible, try to remember what the animal looked like and the area in which you last saw it. Call 9-1-1 or the local emergency number. The dispatcher will get the proper authorities, such as animal control, to the scene.

The stings of some forms of marine life are not only painful but can also make you sick. The side effects include allergic reactions that can cause breathing and heart problems, as well as paralysis. Get trained assistance to remove the person from the water as soon as possible. Call 9-1-1 or the local emergency number if the victim does not know what stung him or her, has a history of allergic reactions to marine life stings, is stung on the face or neck or starts to have trouble breathing.

If you know the sting is from a jellyfish, sea anemone or Portuguese man-of-war, soak the injured part in vinegar as soon as possible. Vinegar works best to offset the toxin, but rubbing alcohol or baking soda may also be used. Do not rub the wound or apply fresh water or ammonia because this increases pain.

If you know the sting is from a sting ray, sea urchin or spiny fish, flush the wound with tap water. Ocean water may also be used. Immobilize the injured part and soak the affected area in non-scalding hot water (as hot as the person can stand) for about 30 minutes or until the pain goes away. If hot water is not available, packing the area in hot sand may have a similar effect if the sand is hot enough. Then carefully clean the wound and apply a bandage. Watch for signs of infection and check with a health-care provider to determine if a tetanus shot is needed.

# ANYONE BITTEN BY AN ANIMAL THAT MIGHT HAVE RABIES MUST GET MEDICAL ATTENTION.

# MOST POISONINGS CAN BE PREVENTED.

## PREVENTING POISONING

Poisoning can be prevented. This is a simple idea, but often people are not careful enough. Use common sense when handling substances that could be harmful, such as chemicals and cleaners. Use them in a well-ventilated area. Wear protective clothing, such as gloves and a face mask.

Use common sense with your own medications. Read the product information and use only as directed. Ask your health-care provider or pharmacist about the intended effects, side effects and possible interactions with other medications you are taking. Never use another person's prescribed medications; what is right for one person is seldom right for another. Always keep medications in the containers they came in and make sure the container is well-marked. Destroy all out-of-date medications by disposing of the contents in the toilet. Over time they can become less effective and even toxic.

---

# HOW TO PREVENT POISONING

**A child can get into trouble in just a moment. Children are curious and can get into things in ways you might not think possible. Almost all child poisonings reported occurred when the child was being watched by a parent or guardian. Many substances found in or around the house are poisonous. Children are especially likely to be poisoned because they tend to put everything into their mouths.**

### Follow these guidelines to guard against poisoning emergencies:

Always supervise children closely, especially in areas where poisons are commonly stored such as in kitchens, bathrooms and garages.

Keep all medications and household products locked away, well out of the reach of children.

Install special clamps to keep children from opening cabinets.

Consider all household or drugstore products to be potentially harmful.

Use childproof safety caps on containers of medication and other potentially dangerous products.

Never call medicine "candy" to get a child to take it, even if it has a pleasant candy flavor.

Read the label.

Keep products in their original containers with the labels in place.

Use poison symbols to identify dangerous substances and teach children what the symbols mean.

Dispose of outdated products as recommended.

Use chemicals only in well-ventilated areas.

During work or recreation that may put you in contact with a poisonous substance, set a good example. Wear proper protective clothing, such as gloves, goggles or a mask.

# How to BEAT those little critters...

You can prevent bites and stings from insects, spiders, ticks or snakes by following these guidelines when you are in wooded or grassy areas.

Wear long-sleeved shirts and long pants.

Tuck your pant legs into your socks or boots.

Tuck your shirt into your pants.

Wear light-colored clothing to make it easier to see tiny insects or ticks.

Use a rubber band or tape to hold pants against socks so that nothing can get under clothing.

When hiking in woods and fields, stay in the middle of trails. Avoid underbrush and tall grass.

If you are outdoors for a long time, check yourself several times during the day. Especially check in hairy areas of the body like the back of the neck and the scalp line.

Inspect yourself carefully for insects or ticks after being outdoors or have someone else do it.

Avoid walking in areas known to be populated with snakes.

If you encounter a snake, look around; there may be others. Turn around and walk away on the same path on which you came.

Wear sturdy hiking boots.

If you have pets that go outdoors, spray them with repellent made for your type of pet. Apply the repellent according to the label and check your pet for ticks often.

If you will be in a grassy or wooded area for a long time, or if you know the area is highly infested with insects or ticks, you may want to use a repellent. (Follow the directions carefully.)

# BATTLING THE

# ENTS

**E**xposure to extreme heat or cold may make a person seriously ill. The likelihood of illness also depends on factors such as physical activity, clothing, wind, humidity, working and living conditions and a person's age and state of mind.

**Temperature, humidity and wind are the three main factors affecting body temperature.**

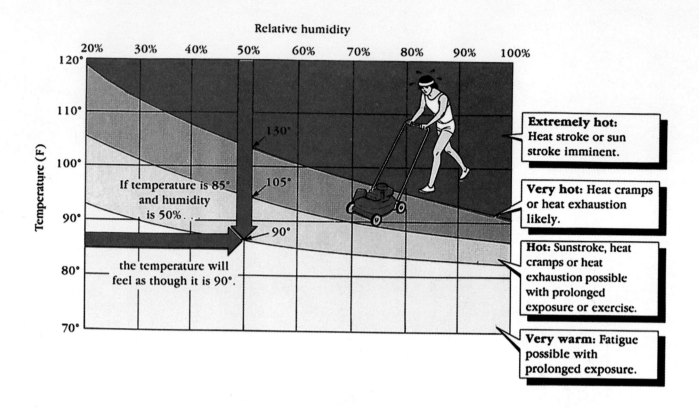

Relative humidity

Extremely hot: Heat stroke or sun stroke imminent.

Very hot: Heat cramps or heat exhaustion likely.

Hot: Sunstroke, heat cramps or heat exhaustion possible with prolonged exposure or exercise.

Very warm: Fatigue possible with prolonged exposure.

If temperature is 85° and humidity is 50%... the temperature will feel as though it is 90°.

Once the signals of a heat- or cold-related illness begin to appear, the victim's condition can quickly get worse. A heat- or cold-related illness can result in death. If you see any of the signals of sudden illness and the victim has been exposed to extremes of heat or cold, suspect a heat- or cold-related illness.

People at risk for heat- or cold-related illnesses include those who work or exercise outdoors, elderly people, young children and people with health problems. Also at risk are those who have had a heat- or cold-related illness in the past, those with medical conditions that cause poor blood circulation and those who take medications to get rid of water from the body (diuretics).

People usually try to get out of extreme heat or cold before they begin to feel ill. However, some people do not or cannot. Athletes and those who work outdoors often keep working even after they begin to feel ill. Those living in buildings that are poorly ventilated, poorly insulated or with poor heating or cooling systems are at increased risk of heat- or cold-related emergencies. Many times, they might not even recognize they are in danger of becoming ill.

## Heat-related Illness

Heat cramps, heat exhaustion and heat stroke are conditions caused by overexposure to heat. Heat cramps are the least severe and often are the first signals that the body is having trouble with the heat. Heat cramps are painful muscle spasms. They usually occur in the legs and abdomen. Think of them as a warning of a possible heat-related emergency.

To care for heat cramps, have the victim rest in a cool place. Give cool water or a commercial sports drink. Usually, rest and fluids are all the person needs to recover. Lightly stretch the muscle and gently massage the area. The victim should not take salt tablets or salt water. They can make the situation worse.

When cramps stop, the person can usually start activity again if there are no other signals of illness. He or she should keep drinking plenty of fluids. Watch the victim carefully for further signals of heat-related illness.

Temperature (F)

**O**nce the signals of a heat- or cold-related illness begin to appear, the victim's condition can quickly become worse.

# Caring For

# HEAT-RELATED ILLNESS

**Resting, lightly stretching the affected muscle and replenishing fluids is usually enough for the body to recover from heat cramps.**

## For Signals of Heat Cramps

- Have the victim move to a cool place.

- Give cool water to drink.

- Have the victim lightly stretch the muscle and gently massage the area.

## For Signals of Heat Exhaustion

- Move the victim to a cooler environment.

- Loosen or remove clothing.

- Fan the victim.

- Get the victim into circulating air while applying water with a cloth or sponge.

- If the victim is conscious, give small amounts of cool water to drink.

- If the victim's condition does not improve or if you suspect heat stroke, call 9-1-1 or the local emergency number.

## For Signals of Heat Stroke

- Call 9-1-1 or the local emergency number.

- Give care until help arrives by following the care steps above for heat exhaustion.

Heat exhaustion is a more severe condition than heat cramps. It often affects athletes, fire fighters, construction workers and factory workers, as well as those who wear heavy clothing in a hot, humid environment. Its signals include cool, moist, pale, ashen or flushed skin; headache; nausea; dizziness; weakness; and exhaustion.

Heat stroke is the least common but most severe heat emergency. It most often occurs when people ignore the signals of heat exhaustion. Heat stroke develops when the body systems are overwhelmed by heat and begin to stop functioning. Heat stroke is a serious medical emergency. The signals of heat stroke include red skin that can be either dry or moist; changes in consciousness; rapid, weak pulse; and rapid, shallow breathing.

When you recognize heat-related illness in its early stages, you can usually reverse it. Get the victim out of the heat. Loosen any tight clothing and apply cool, wet cloths, such as towels or sheets, taking care to remoisten the cloths periodically. Spraying the victim with 100 percent water and fanning is also beneficial. If the victim is conscious, give him or her small amounts of cool water to drink.

Do not let the conscious victim drink too quickly. Give about one glass (4 ounces) of water every 15 minutes. Let the victim rest in a comfortable position and watch carefully for changes in his or her condition. The victim should not resume normal activities the same day.

Refusing water, vomiting and changes in consciousness mean that the victim's condition is getting worse. Call 9-1-1 or the local emergency number immediately if you have not already done so. If the victim vomits, stop giving fluids and place the victim on his or her side. Watch for signals of breathing problems. Keep the victim lying down and continue to cool the body any way you can. If you have ice packs or cold packs, place them on each of the victim's wrists and ankles, on the groin, in each armpit and on the neck to cool the large blood vessels. Use barriers, like towels or clothing, between the ice packs and the victim to protect the skin. *Do not* apply rubbing (isopropyl) alcohol.

**To cool the body of a victim of heat-related illness, cover with cool, wet towels and apply cold packs, if necessary.**

**R**efusing water, vomiting and changes in consciousness mean that the victim's condition is getting worse.

## Cold-related Illness

Frostbite and hypothermia are two types of cold-related emergencies. Frostbite is the freezing of body parts exposed to the cold. Severity depends on the air temperature, length of exposure and the wind. Frostbite can cause the loss of fingers, hands, arms, toes, feet and legs.

The signals of frostbite include lack of feeling in the affected area and skin that appears waxy, is cold to the touch or is discolored (flushed, white, yellow or blue).

To care for any frostbite, handle the area gently. Never rub an affected area. Rubbing causes further damage to soft tissues. Instead, warm the area gently by soaking the affected part in water not warmer than 105° F. If you do not have a thermometer, test the water temperature yourself. If the temperature is uncomfortable to your touch, the water is too warm. Keep the frostbitten part in the water until it looks red and feels warm. Loosely bandage the area with a dry, sterile dressing. If fingers or toes are frostbitten, place cotton or gauze between them. Do not break any blisters. Get emergency medical help as soon as possible.

In hypothermia the entire body cools because its ability to keep warm fails. The victim will die if not given care. Signals of hypothermia include shivering,

**T**he air temperature does not have to be below freezing for someone to get hypothermia.

numbness, glassy stare, apathy and loss of consciousness.

The air temperature does not have to be below freezing for people to develop hypothermia. Elderly people in poorly heated homes can develop hypothermia at higher temperatures. The homeless and the ill also are at risk. Substances that interfere with the body's normal response to cold, such as alcohol, may cause hypothermia to occur more easily. Any medical condition that impairs circulation, such as diabetes or cardiovascular disease, can also make a person more likely to get hypothermia. Anyone remaining in cold water or wet clothing for a long time may also easily develop hypothermia.

To care for hypothermia, start by caring for any life-threatening conditions. Call 9-1-1 or the local emergency number. Make the victim comfortable. Remove any wet clothing and dry the victim. Warm the body gradually by wrapping the victim in blankets or putting on dry clothing and moving him or her to a warm place. If they are available, apply heat pads or other heat sources to the body.

Keep a barrier, such as a blanket, towel or clothing, between the heat source and the victim to avoid burning him or her. If the victim is alert, give warm liquids to drink. Do not warm the victim too quickly, such as by immersing the victim in warm water. Rapid rewarming can cause dangerous heart problems. Handle the victim gently.

In cases of severe hypothermia, the victim may be unconscious. Breathing might have slowed or stopped. The pulse may be slow and irregular. In these circumstances, when checking for signs of circulation, the pulse should be checked for up to 30 to 45 seconds. The body may feel stiff because the muscles become rigid. Call 9-1-1 or the local emergency number. Keep checking breathing and signs of circulation. Give rescue breathing if necessary. Continue to warm the victim until EMS personnel arrive. Be prepared to start CPR and use an AED, if appropriate.

In general, illnesses caused by overexposure to extreme temperatures can be prevented. To prevent heat- and cold-related emer-

100-105°F

**To care for frostbite, warm the frostbitten area by soaking the area in water *(left)*. Do not allow the frostbitten area to touch the container. After rewarming, bandage the area with dry, sterile dressings. If fingers or toes are frostbitten, place gauze between them *(right)*.**

gencies from happening to you or anyone you know, follow these guidelines:

- Avoid being outdoors in the hottest or coldest part of the day.
- Change your activity level according to the temperatures.
- Take frequent breaks.
- Dress appropriately for the environment.
- Drink large amounts of fluids.

For a hypothermia victim, rewarm the body gradually by wrapping the victim in blankets or putting on dry clothing and moving him or her to a warm place.

Taking frequent breaks when exercising in extreme temperatures allows your body to readjust to normal body temperature.

## Caring For
# COLD-RELATED ILLNESS

### For Signals of Hypothermia

- Gently move the victim to a warm place.
- Check ABCs and care for shock.
- Remove wet clothing and cover the victim with blankets and plastic sheeting to hold in body heat.
- Carefully monitor use of heating pads and hot water bottles so that the victim is not unintentionally burned.
- Warm the victim slowly and handle the victim carefully.

### For Frostbite

- Remove wet clothing and jewelry from the affected area.
- Soak the frostbitten area in warm water.
- Cover with dry, sterile dressings—do not rub the frostbitten area.
- Check ABCs and care for shock.
- Do not rewarm a frostbitten part if there is a danger of it refreezing.

# The High-Tech War Against Cold

In the past, we depended entirely on nature for clothing. Animal skins, furs and feathers protected us from freezing temperatures. As long as seasonal changes and cold climates exist, preventing cold-related illnesses, such as hypothermia, remains important when we work or play outside. Although natural fibers, such as wool and down, are still very useful, a whole family of synthetic fibers is now used to make clothing. Being outdoors has become a lot more comfortable.

The best way to use outdoor fabrics is to layer them. This creates warmth by trapping warm air between layers to insulate the body. Layering is an old concept: wear several layers of clothing when it's cold; take clothes off when warm and put them back on if you get cold. This enables you to regulate your body temperature and deal with changes in the environment.

Start off with an underwear or base layer. Commonly called long underwear, it includes thin, snug-fitting pants and a long-sleeved shirt. Underwear should supply you with basic insulation and pull moisture away from your skin—damp, sweaty skin can chill you when you slow down or stop activity. Natural fibers, such as cotton, wool and silk, can be quite warm and are okay for light activity. For heavier exercise, however, synthetic fabrics absorb less moisture and actually carry water droplets away from your skin. Polypropylene™, Thermax™ and Capilene™ are popular synthetic fabrics for underwear.

Next, add one or more insulating layers, such as a wool sweater or a polyester fleece or down jacket, depending on the temperature. Do not forget your legs. Wool, non-cotton or fleece pants are a better choice than jeans or corduroys. Synthetic materials used in jackets and pants include Thinsulate™, Qualofil™ and pile (a plush, nonpiling polyester

fiber). Although down is an excellent, lightweight insulator, it becomes useless when wet, so a quick-drying, fabric-like pile may keep you warmer in a damp climate.

Finish with a windproof, and preferably waterproof, shell layer. Synthetic, high-tech fabrics make a strong showing here. Some shell layers are waterproof and windproof, but not breathable. These are made of polyester and/or nylon with a polyurethane coating. High-tech fabrics can be windproof, waterproof and breathable. Those are usually nylon fabrics treated with a breathable, waterproof membrane such as EncapSil™ or Gore-Tex®.

Layering clothing allows the wearer to regulate body temperature and deal with changes in weather. Clothing layers can be used in combination or separately, depending on the climate and activity.

## Inner Layer

Recreational Equipment Inc.

**Capilene**  Lightweight, synthetic fabric that doesn't absorb moisture. Designed to pull moisture away from skin where it can evaporate.

**Cotton**  Soft, natural fibers that absorb moisture and allow air to circulate.

## Insulating Layer

**Qualofil**  Exceptionally warm, wet or dry.

**Pile**  Soft, polyester fabric that is warmer per pound than wool. Insulates when wet and is quick drying.

## Shell Layer

**Ripstop Nylon**  Windproof, resistant to moisture, and has some breathability. Protects against fog, light rain and snow.

**Hypalon**  Versatile, synthetic rubber applied to lightweight nylon is completely water repellent. Unaffected by saltwater and highly resistant to abrasion.

**Supplex**  Lightweight nylon that is cotton-soft yet strong. Windproof, breathable, some water repellency and quick drying.

**Gore-Tex**  Is used in combination with water-repellent exterior fabric. Allows perspiration to escape while preventing water and wind from seeping in.

231

# THE YOUNG AND THE ELDERLY

**C**aring for an ill or injured child is not always easy, especially if it is a child you do not know. Children are not simply small adults. They have unique needs and require special care. Some children do not readily accept strangers. This can make it difficult to accurately check a child's condition. Young children can be especially difficult to check, since they often will not be able to tell you what is wrong.

It is often difficult to imagine how a young child with a serious

illness or injury feels. One of a child's main emotions is fear. The fears that a child experiences are real. A child is afraid of the unknown. He or she is afraid of being ill or hurt, of being touched by strangers and of being separated from his or her parents. How you interact with a child is very important. You need to try to reduce anxiety and panic in the child.

Children up to 1 year of age are commonly referred to as infants. Young infants, those less than 6 months old, are relatively easy to approach. Your presence will not generally bother children of this age group. Older infants,

# Kids have unique needs that require special care.

however, will often exhibit "stranger anxiety." They are uncomfortable around strangers and may cry and cling to a parent or guardian.

Children 1 to 3 years of age are called toddlers. These children are frequently uncooperative. A toddler will be concerned that he or she will be separated

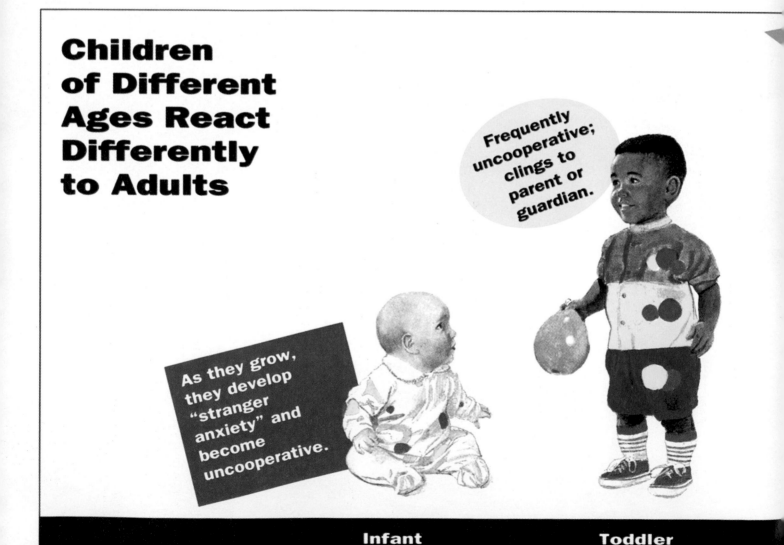

# Children of Different Ages React Differently to Adults

Frequently uncooperative; clings to parent or guardian.

As they grow, they develop "stranger anxiety" and become uncooperative.

Infant
0-1

Toddler
1-3

from the parent or guardian. Reassurance that this will not happen will often comfort a concerned child of this age. It is often best to check a toddler in the parent or guardian's lap.

Children 3 to 5 are generally referred to as preschoolers. Children in this age group are usually easy to check if approached properly. Use their natural curiosity. Allow them to inspect items such as bandages.

School-aged children are 5 to 13 years of age. They are usually cooperative and can be a good source of information about what happened. You should be able to talk with them readily. Children in this age group are becoming conscious of their bodies. Respect the child's modesty.

Adolescents are 13 to 18 years of age. They are typically more like an adult than a child. Direct your questions to them instead of to parents or guardians. However, allow input from a parent or guardian. Occasionally, in the presence of a parent or guardian, it may not be possible to get an accurate idea of what happened or what is wrong. Also adolescents are modest and often respond better to a caregiver of the same gender.

## Kids Have Special Problems

Injury remains the number one cause of death for children in

Usually cooperative; naturally curious.

Usually cooperative; able to get information from them.

Modest; usually responds better to a caregiver of the same gender. Normally cooperative.

**Preschooler 3-5**

**School-age 5-13**

**Adolescent 13-18**

**Because a child's head is usually large in proportion to the body, the head is often injured.**

the United States. Many of these deaths are the result of motor vehicle accidents. The greatest dangers to a child involved in a vehicle incident that results in serious injury are a blocked airway and bleeding. Because a child's head is usually large in proportion to the rest of the body, the head is often injured.

To avoid some of the needless deaths of children associated with motor vehicles, laws have been enacted requiring that children ride in car seats or use safety belts, as appropriate. As a result, more lives will be saved.

You may have to check and care for an injured child while he or she is in a car seat. A car seat does not normally pose any problem when you are trying to check a child. A child involved in a motor vehicle accident and found in a car seat should be left in the seat if the device has not been damaged. If the child is to be transported to a medical facility for evaluation, he or she can be easily secured in the car seat.

A high fever in a child indicates some type of infection. In a young child, even a minor infection can result in a rather high fever. This is often defined as a temperature above 103° F. Prolonged or excessively high fever can result in seizures. Your initial care for a child with high fever is to gently cool the child. This includes removing excessive clothing or blankets and sponging lukewarm water on the child. Call the child's health-care provider at once.

Infections that affect breathing are more common in children than adults. These can range from minor infections, such as the common cold, to life-threatening infections that block the airway.

One such illness is croup.

Croup is an infection that causes swelling of the throat below the vocal cords. Besides the basic signals of breathing problems and a cough that sounds like the bark of a seal, croup is often preceded by 1 or 2 days of illness, sometimes with a fever. Croup occurs more often in the winter months and the signals are often evident in the evening. It generally is not life threatening. The child will often improve when exposed to cool air, such as air outdoors or cool steam from a vaporizer.

Another childhood problem is epiglottitis. This is an infection that causes a severe inflammation of the epiglottis, a flap of tissue above the vocal cords that protects the airway during swallowing. When it becomes infected, the epiglottis can swell to a point where the airway is completely blocked. The child with epiglottitis will appear quite ill and have a high fever. He or she will often be sitting up and straining to breathe. The child will be very frightened. Saliva may be drooling from his or her mouth because swelling of the epiglottis prevents the child from swallowing.

You will not need to distinguish between croup and epiglottitis, since the care you provide will be the same for either situation. To care for a child who is having trouble breathing, allow him or her to remain in the most comfortable position for breathing. Do not attempt to place any objects in the child's mouth. Call the child's health-care provider at once. If this is not possible, call 9-1-1 or your local emergency number. If the child's airway becomes completely blocked as a result of epiglottitis, there is nothing you can do to help; this child needs professional help **immediately.** Call 9-1-1 or

# CHECKING A CHILD

**Checking an ill or injured child can be a challenge, especially if you do not know him or her. The following are a few basic guidelines that will help you.**

### Observe the Child Before Touching Him or Her

You can find out much information before you actually touch the child. Look for signals that indicate changes in consciousness, any trouble breathing and any apparent injuries or conditions. All may change as soon as you touch the child because he or she may become anxious or upset.

### Remain Calm

Caring for ill or injured children can be very stressful. Staying calm will show confidence and help keep the child and parent or guardian calm.

### Communicate Clearly with the Parent or Guardian and the Child

If the family is excited or agitated, the child is likely to be so too. When you can calm the family, the child will often calm down as well. Explain what you wish to do. Get at eye level with the child. Talk slowly and use simple words when speaking with the child. Ask questions that can be easily answered.

### Do Not Separate the Child from Loved Ones Unless Necessary

This is especially true for younger children (under age 7 or 8). Often a parent or guardian will be holding a crying child. In this case, you can check the child while the parent or guardian continues to hold him or her.

### Gain Trust Through Your Actions

Explain what you are going to do before you do it. Be sure to use terms and language the child will understand. Check a conscious child from the feet to the head rather than head to toe. The child is more likely to accept you first touching the feet and progressing to the head. You should still look and feel for the same things.

the local emergency number immediately.

## Older Adults

The elderly are generally considered those 65 years of age and older. They are the fastest growing population group in the United States. A major reason is an increase in life expectancy because of improvements in health care. Since 1900, there

**MEMO**

*"Joe, I'm really beginning to worry about your dad. At first it was just little things—like forgetting where he put his glasses and what day it was and how to work the VCR, but now it's worse. Last week he went out and Mrs. Chung found him wandering the street and brought him home. He couldn't remember where he lived or who he was! Yesterday, he just walked out while we were talking. Later, he didn't remember anything about it. It's not safe for him to be out by himself anymore. Maybe there's something that will make him better. I just don't know what I'm going to do!"*

Joe's dad needs several medical examinations to try to determine the reasons for his memory decline. Perhaps he has a condition that can be reversed or helped. But the chances are high that he has a condition known as Alzheimer's disease. At one time considered a rare disorder, today Alzheimer's disease (AD) (pronounced awlz-heimer's) is a progressive disease characterized by memory loss, language deterioration, impaired visual skills, poor judgment and an indifferent attitude, but retained motor abilities.[80] Dementia is the loss of intellectual functions such as thinking, remembering and reasoning, that is severe enough to interfere with a person's daily activities.

AD affects an estimated 4 million American adults. A person lives with Alzheimer's an average of 8 years and as many as 20 years or more from the onset of signals.[81] Neither Medicare nor private health insurance covers the type of comprehensive long-term care most victims need. Those with Alzheimer's disease generally are over 65; however, AD can strike people in their 40s and 50s. Men and women are affected almost equally. At this time, scientists are still looking for the cause of AD. A confirmed diagnosis of the disease can only be made by examining the victim's brain tissue after death. And while there are no treatments to stop or reverse the mental decline from AD, several drugs are available now to help manage some of the signals.

Signals of AD develop gradually. They include confusion, progressive memory loss and changes in personality, behavior and the ability to think and communicate. Eventually, victims of AD become totally unable to care for themselves.

has been a 55 percent increase in life expectancy. For example, in 1900, the average life expectancy was 49 years. Today the average life expectancy is over 76 years.[79]

Many changes occur with age. Overall, there is general decline in body function, with some changes beginning as early as age 30. Both the heart and the lungs suffer the effects of aging. The

There are a number of disorders that have symptoms similar to those of AD. Some of them can be treated. Therefore, it is very important that anyone who is experiencing memory loss or confusion has a thorough medical examination.

Most people with illnesses such as AD are cared for by their families for much of their illness. Providing care at home requires careful planning. The home has to be made safe and routines set up for daily activities such as mealtimes, personal care and leisure.

**Services That Help**

It is important for anyone caring for a person with Alzheimer's or a related problem to realize that they are not alone. There are people and organizations that can help both you and the person with AD. Your health-care provider can give you medical advice, including help with difficult behavior and personality changes.

If you are caring for an AD victim living at home, you may need help with some basic services such as nutrition and transportation. A visiting nurse or nutritionist can help you and a volunteer program like Meals on Wheels may be helpful. Volunteer or paid transportation services may also be available to take AD victims to and from health facilities, adult day care, respite services and other programs.

Visiting nurses, home health aides and homemakers can come to your home and provide help with health care, bathing and dressing, shopping and cooking. Many adult day care centers provide recreational activities designed for

people with AD. Some hospitals, nursing homes and other facilities may take in AD victims for short stays. For AD victims who can no longer live at home, group homes or foster homes may be available. Nursing homes offer more skilled nursing and some specialize in the care of victims of AD or similar diseases. A few hospice programs accept AD victims who are nearing the end of their life. Explore to find out which, if any, services are covered by Medicare, Medicaid, Social Security disability or veterans' benefits in your state. A lawyer or a social worker may be able to help you.

To locate services that can help you, the AD victim and other family members, check the yellow pages under Social Service Organizations and state and local government listings in the phone directory. Places you can call for information include your local health department, area agency on aging and department of social services or senior citizen's services. Churches, synagogues and other religious institutions may also have information and programs; so may senior centers and nursing home staffs, hospital geriatric departments, doctors, nurses, social workers and counselors. Your location may have a chapter of the Alzheimer's Association nearby. To locate a chapter near you, call the **Alzheimer's Association's toll-free number: 1-800-272-3900 between 8 a.m. and 5 p.m. CST.** This organization has chapters and support groups across the country where you can get information and guidance.

# Older adults are more prone to injury and illness as body functions generally decline.

amount of blood pumped by the heart with each beat decreases and the heart rate slows. The blood vessels harden, causing increased work for the heart. The number of working brain cells also decreases with age. Hearing and vision usually decline, often causing some degree of sight and hearing loss. Reflexes become slower and arthritis may affect joints, causing movement to become painful.

As a result of slower reflexes, failing eyesight and hearing, arthritis and problems related to the blood vessels, such as numbness, the elderly are at increased risk of injury from falls. Falls frequently result in fractures because the bones become weaker and more brittle with age.

An elderly person is also at greater risk of serious head injuries. This is mainly because as we age, the size of the brain decreases. This results in more space between the surface of the brain and the inside of the skull, which can increase the likelihood of serious head injury. Occasionally, an elderly person may not develop the signals of a head injury until days after a fall. Therefore, you should always suspect a head injury as a possible cause of unusual behavior in an elderly person, especially if the victim has had a fall or blow to the head.

The elderly are also prone to problems with the nervous system, especially stroke. In addition, the elderly are at increased risk of altered thinking patterns and confusion. Some change is a result of aging. However, certain diseases occurring in some elderly persons also cause problems with the way the mind works. The most common of these is Alzheimer's disease, a disease that affects the brain. It results in impaired memory, thinking and behavior. Alzheimer's affects an estimated 4 million adults.

If you are providing care for an elderly person who is confused, try to find out whether the confusion is a result of injury or a condition the victim already has. Get at the victim's eye level so that he or she can see and hear you more clearly. Sometimes confusion is actually the result of decreased vision or hearing.

Your care for the elderly victim requires you to keep in mind the special problems and concerns of the elderly and to communicate appropriately. Often, an elderly victim's problem will seem unimportant to him or her. He or she may not recognize the signals of a serious condition. The victim may also downplay signals out of fear of losing his or her independence or of being placed in a nursing home. Do not talk down to an elderly person, as you would a child. In some circumstances, you should gather the victim's medications and see that they are with the victim if he or she is being taken to a medical facility.